# Classical Chinese Medicine Made Visible

# 图说经典中医

Dr. Pan, Xiaochuan

潘晓川

# CONTENTS

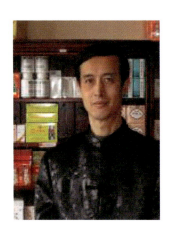

ISBN-10: 1482340712
ISBN-13: 978-1482340716

Dr. Pan

# PREFACE

Heaven, Earth and Human are three vitals in our universe. "Human takes laws from the Earth; the Earth follows Heaven; Heaven follows the Dao; and the Dao is the source" (Lao Zi). In turn, the Dao and these universal laws apply to us as humans. This is Classical Chinese Medicine.

Chinese medicine originated from Heaven above. Evidence can be found in both ancient and modern astrology for almost all of these basic concepts. The more we know about the universe, the more amazed we are in the truth of ancient wisdom.

This book is meant to be viewed more than read. Pictures and diagrams are used in this book to make Classical Chinese Medicine visible through the Yi Jing. The purpose is to set up the symbolic image and numerology model that was the original way of thinking for Chinese Medicine in ancient times.

# About This Book

I am incredibly grateful for the wisdom Dr. Pan has shared with me personally, and also for all those who will have the same chance through studying this book.

The material presented herein represents the same methodology of thought that was the foundation of the Chinese Medicine Classics. Likewise, it is also transmitted in the traditional way, using few words but a multitude of symbolism and imagery.

As the ancient sages would have, when we look to the stars, to heaven, to nature, to the earth and at ourselves we start to see similarities and cycles of movement that pervade throughout. Through contemplating these correlations and relationships we begin to develop much deeper meanings and understandings. Then, in the spirit of the Dao, even the greatest complexity can be made extremely simple.

By contemplating the information within this book you will never look at Chinese Medicine the same way again. You may not even look at life the same way again! Whether you are an acupuncturist, an herbalist or a scholar, it will answer many questions, and hopefully it will stimulate many more.

It is a very exciting time for Chinese Medicine and I feel very blessed to share in the many gifts the Classics have to offer. Thankfully there are books like this to light the way.

David Arnold

# 1 THE KNOWN UNIVERSE

What were the requirements in the Inner Cannon for Chinese medicine doctors? "To be a doctor, one must know the heaven above, the Earth below, and the human in the middle." The reason for this is that Chinese medicine applies the laws of the universe to the human body. The ancient people knew those laws by observing the sky, Earth, and comparing human beings to all other things in the world.

How can a person know so much about the heaven and the Earth? It has to be through learning Yi Jing. "Yi Jing covers everything, the laws of heaven, the Earth and the human. Three divided into six becomes a hexagram which symbolizes the three vitals of heaven, Earth and the human." Yi Jing is the philosophy of Classical Chinese Medicine.

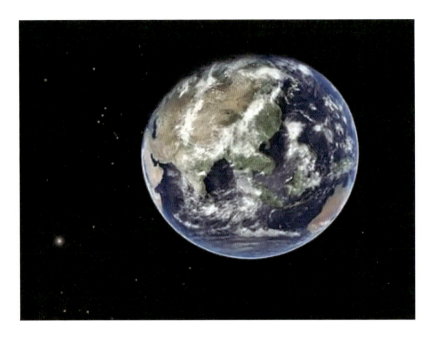

What does the universe look like? Let's follow the telescope, and start our journey from the Earth, our sweet home.

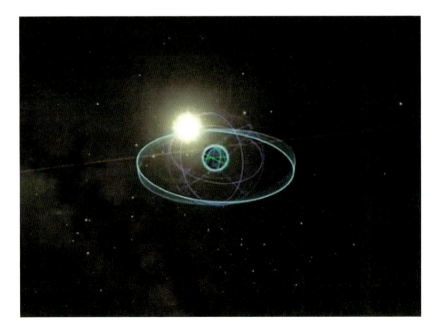

View from the distance of one second light travel time from Earth

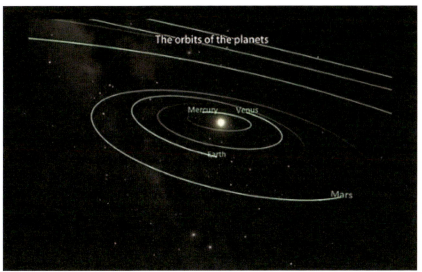

One hour light travel time from Earth: Solar system. Five stars named by wood, fire, Earth, metal and water according to their colors. Together with the Sun and Moon, there were 7 administrative stars.

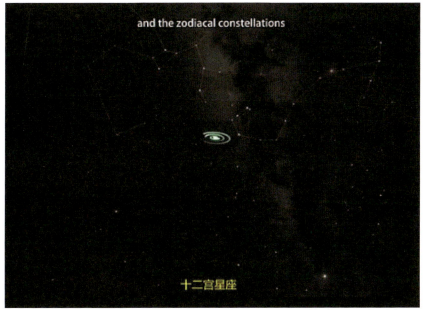

One day light travel time from Earth; 28 Constellations of Chinese Ancient astrology were divided into 4 groups with 7 in each group.

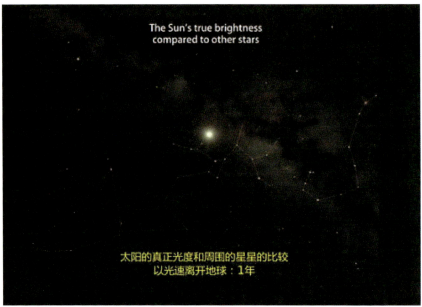

1 light year from Earth

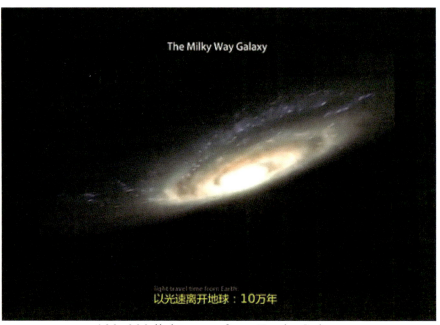

100, 000 light years from Earth: Galaxy

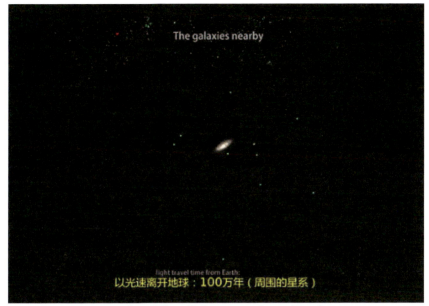

1 million light years from Earth

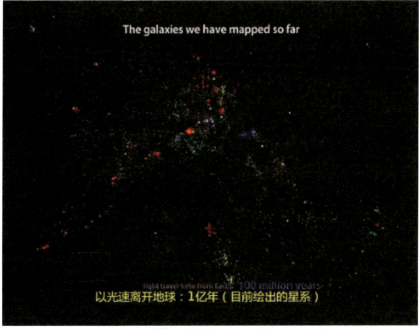

100 million light years from Earth

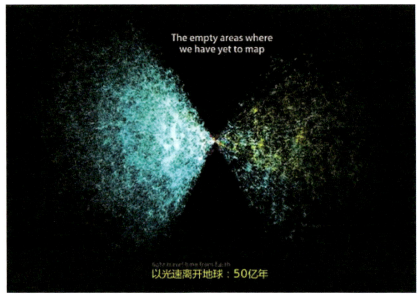

5 billion light years from the Earth: The largest double spiral structure known to mankind.

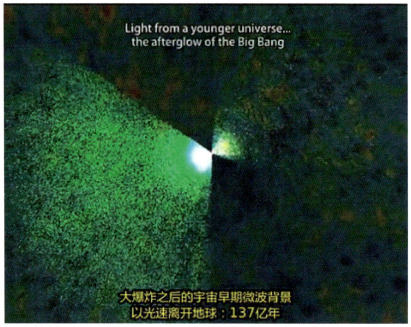

13.7 billion years light years from Earth: One spiral is the material universe and the other one is the antimatter universe. The connection part is the so-called "Black Hole".

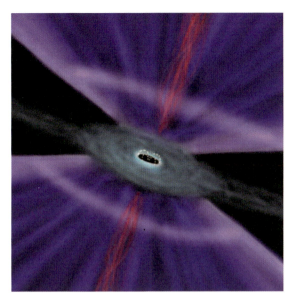

Light from the material universe travels though the Black Hole to the antimatter universe. From our side of the universe, the connection part looks black, so we call it "Black Hole". On the other side of the universe, the light bursts out, looks very bight, so it is called "White Hole".

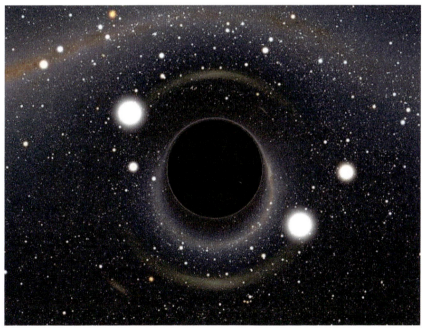

Black Hole is the creator of the universe. Before the Big Bang, there was "nothing" but energy. Our material universe came from the explosion. Eventually, the Black Hole will swallow everything and back to "nothing" again and finish one big universal breath.

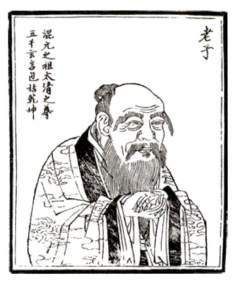

Lao Zi (5th–4th century BCE) described this Black Hole as "Dao" in "Dao De Jing":

"有物混成，先天地生。
寂兮寥兮，独立而不改，
周行而不殆，可以为天下母。
吾不知其名，强字之曰道"

"There was something formless and perfect before the universe was born. It is serene. Empty. Solitary. Unchanging. Infinite. Eternally present. It is the mother of the universe. For lack of a better name, I call it the Dao."

In Buddhism, it is believed that souls exist forever. After death, souls go to different spaces according to what they did in this world. What do we know about near-death experience in the West?

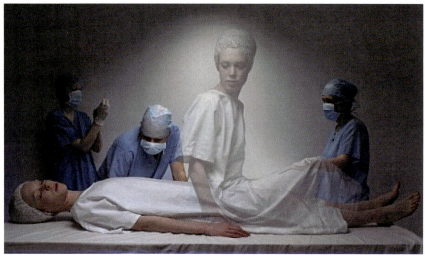

Leave the body and watch the body from above

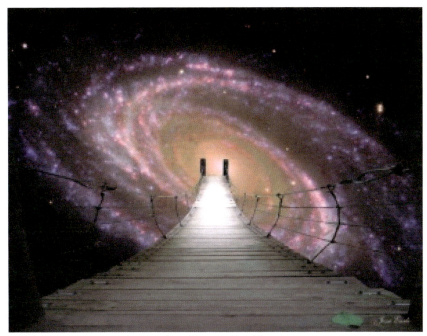

Floating to the Sky

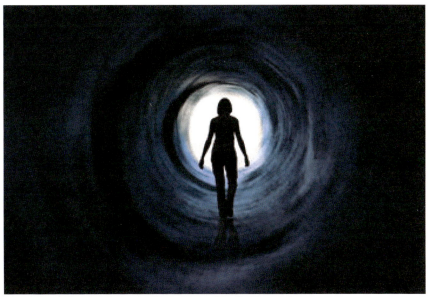

Passing a Dark Tunnel

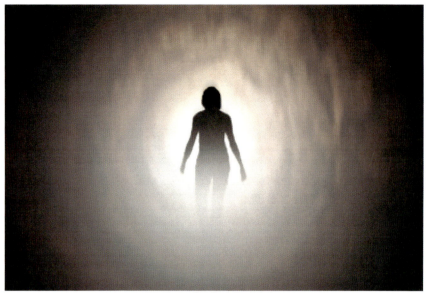

Go into the Bright Light

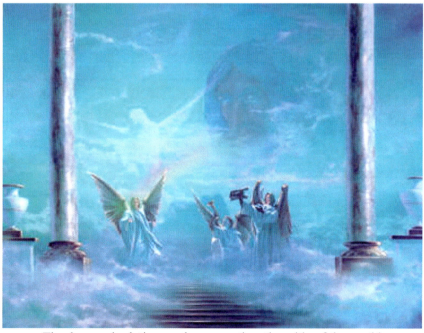

The deceased relatives welcome on the other side of the world

# 2 TAIJI, THE 3 DIMENSION MODEL OF THE UNIVERSE

Taiji is the symbol of Chinese medicine. Not only that, Taiji is also the 3 dimension model of the universe. It is also the basic structure and movement for all in this material world. The sage in the ancient times must have known this or they would not have written like this: "道可道，非常道；名可名，非常名"。"Dao that can be described is not universal and eternal Dao. The name that can be named is not the enduring and unchanging name."

Suppose let's go back to the time a few thousand years ago. Based on the most recent discoveries on astrology, how would you tell the people at that time? I am afraid you still have to say like Lao Tzu: The universe is too complicated to describe. If I say it, it is not itself any more. If I name it, then it is not the right thing I want to tell you. So I have to create a word for it: Dao.

How those sages know the truth of the universe? By internal discovery, that is meditation. Practioners in Daoism or Buddhism found the same thing and the records were quite the same. This was the true origin of Chinese medicine.

And the ancient records are quite the same to the external discoveries as pictures we just watched.

# Black and White Holes

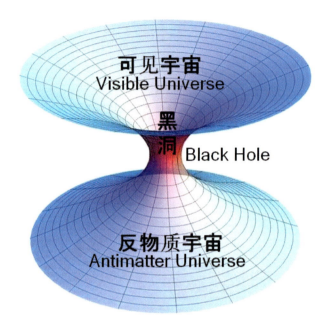

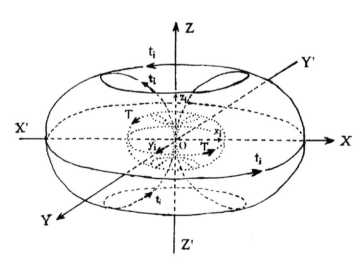

Black Hole: Mathematic Model of 11 Dimensions

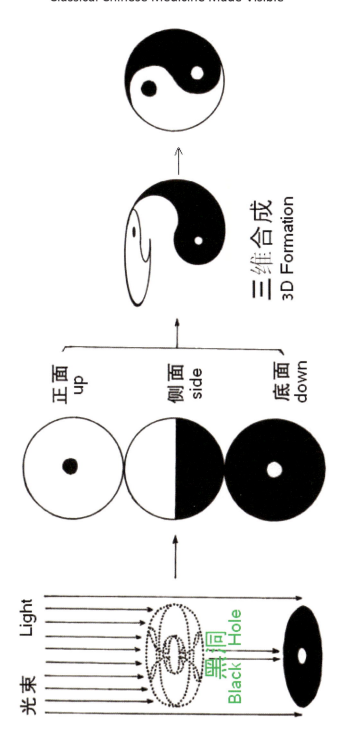

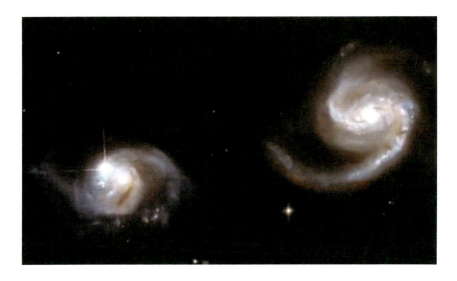

Merging of Two Galaxies

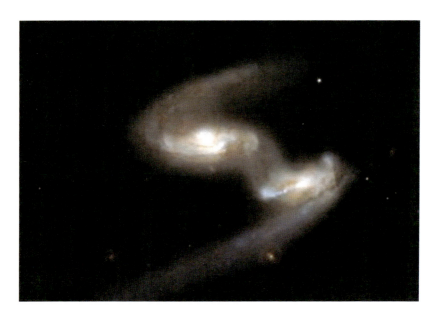

Two Wings

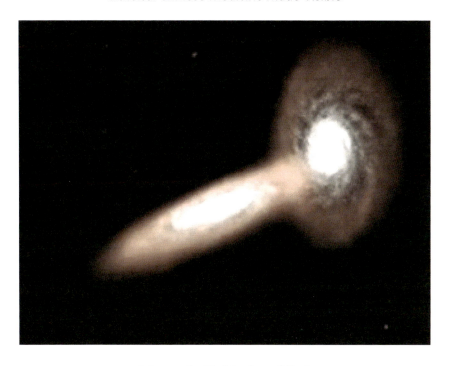

Magnetic Fields Amplified

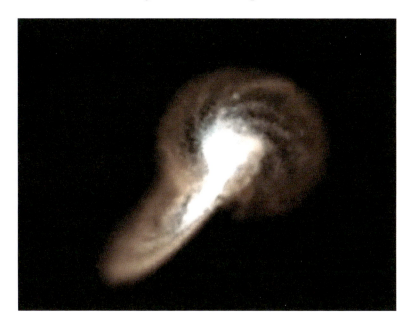

Matter Evacuated

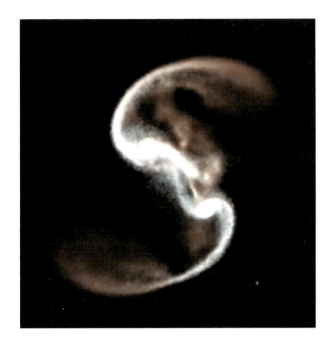

Funnel Structure

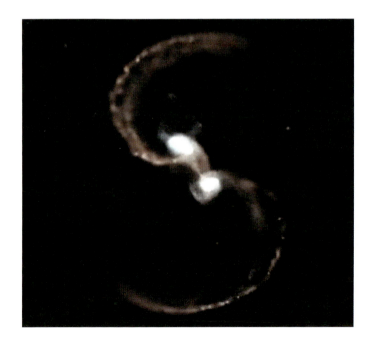

Double Spiral

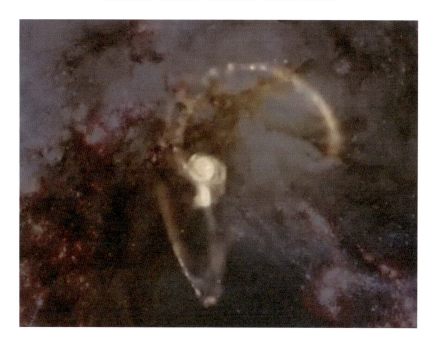

Merged Black Hole

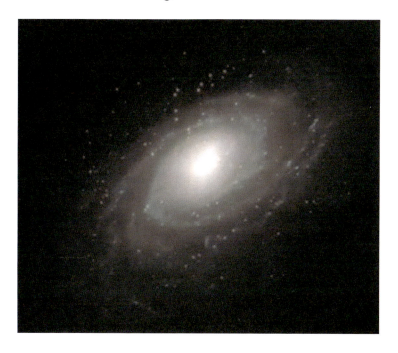

Accretion Disk

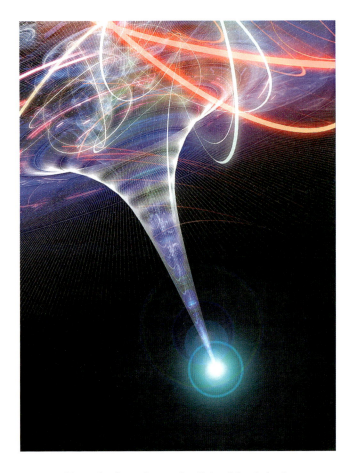

Singularity, the end of the black hole

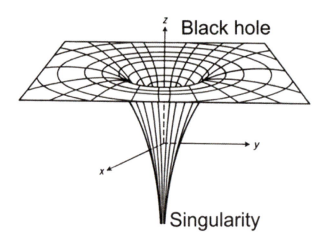

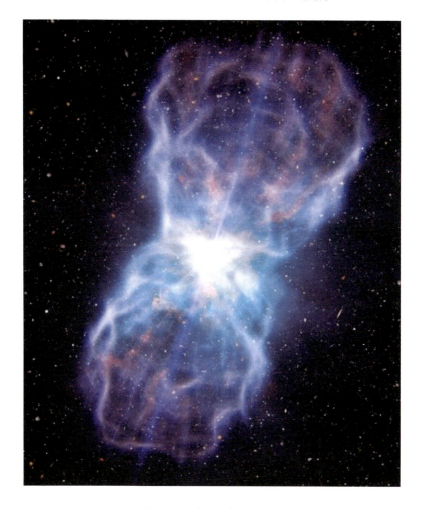

Quasar, the white hole

Quasars are believed to be the so called "white holes" powered by accretion of material into supermassive black holes in the nuclei of distant galaxies, making these luminous versions of the general class of objects known as active galaxies.

When matter from the singularity of a black hole and anti-matter from the singularity from the white hole merge together, both matters swallow each other, matters disappear and great energy is created, another "Big Bang" happens again and a new double spiral universe is borne. That is the Life Cycle of Universes.

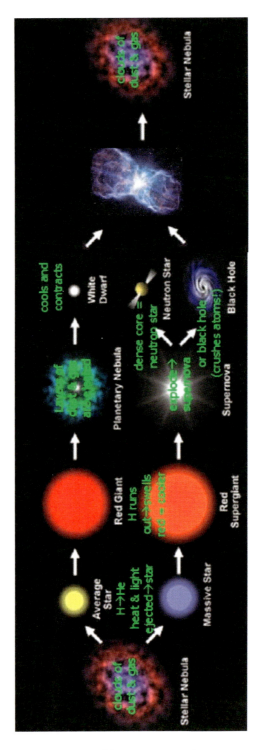

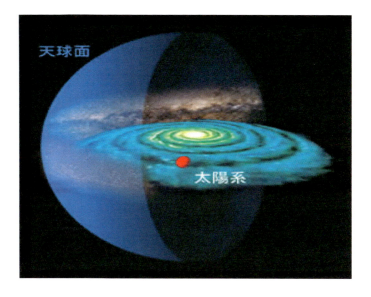

Chinese Ancient theory of the universe: The heaven is like an Egg

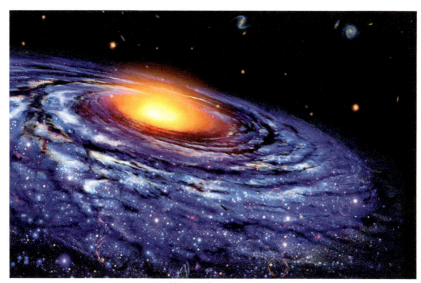

Taiji: Solar System

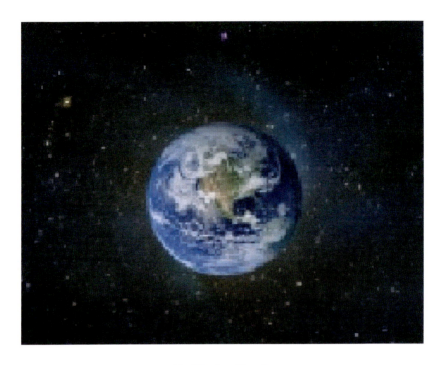

Taiji: the Earth

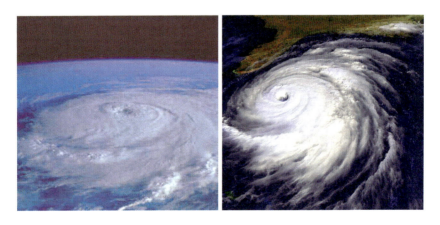

Taiji: Atmosphere          Taiji: Hurricane

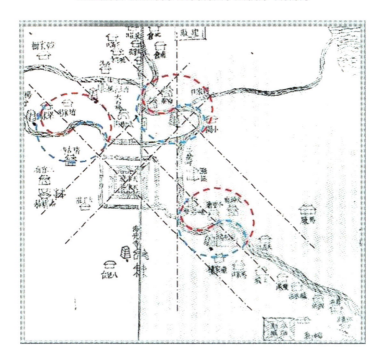

Tianjin city held by 3 Taiji

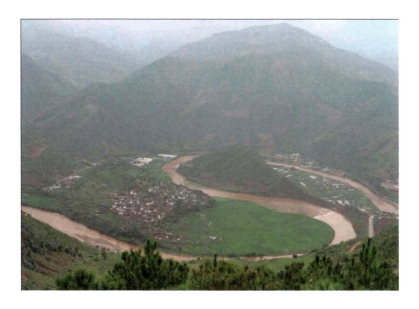

Natural Taiji in Dali, China

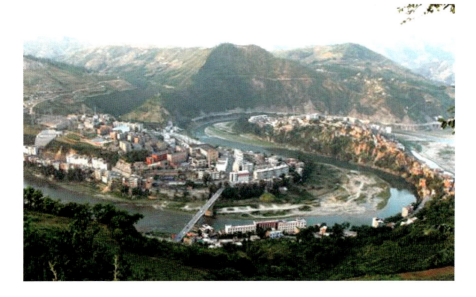

Natural Taiji in Shaanxi, China

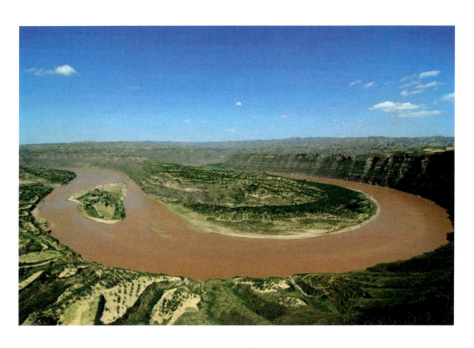

One Curve of Yellow River

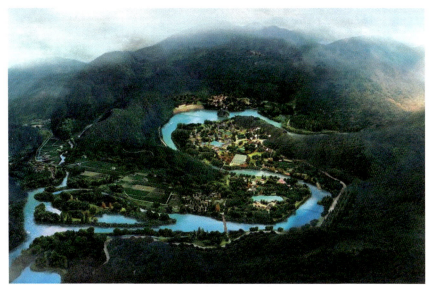

Ru He Village, China

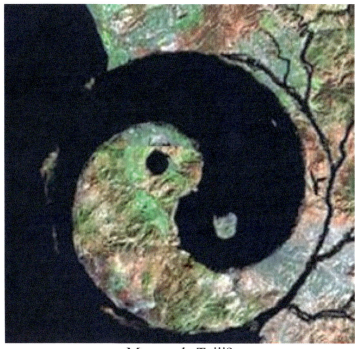

Man made Taiji?

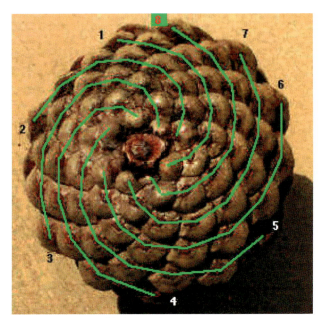

Beautiful Work of the Nature

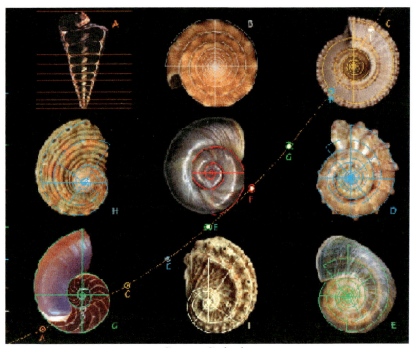

Secret Spirals

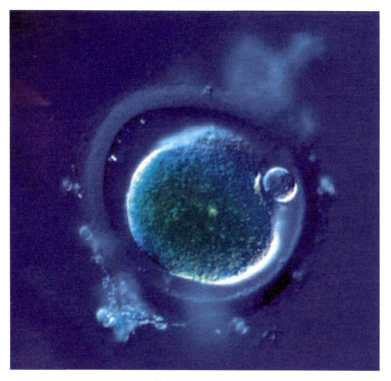

Taiji: Human Egg

"在天成像，在地成形". "Image over the sky, shape on the Earth". It really happened.

More than 2 thousand crop circles were found since 1970. Now it is still world mystery to human kind. Some researchers believe they are related to UFO's and alien beings. It might be the communications from among stars.

It is said crop circles are formed very quickly. One pilot reported that a crop circle had formed within the half an hour of his returning flight. One researcher video taped the formation of one crop circle. Two lights from the sky turning around and the circle was done in a few minutes while there was nothing you could see in the sky above them.

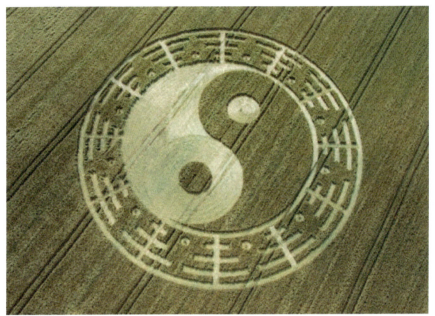

United Kingdom, Stantonbury Hill, N. Somerset, 7 July 2007

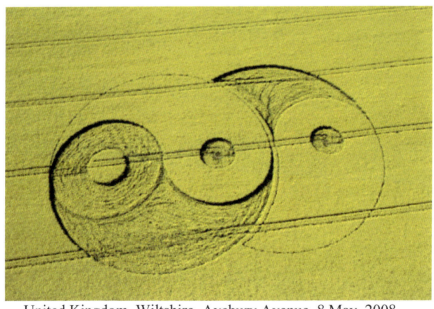

United Kingdom, Wiltshire, Avebury Avenue, 8 May, 2008

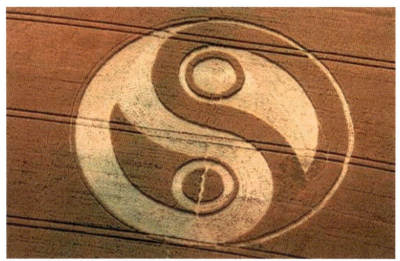

Germany, 07 July, 2008

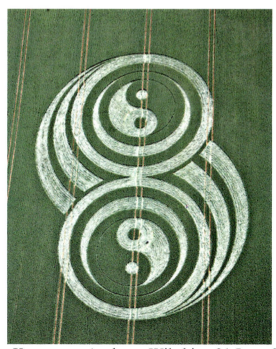

West Kennett, nr Avebury, Wiltshire, 21 June, 2009

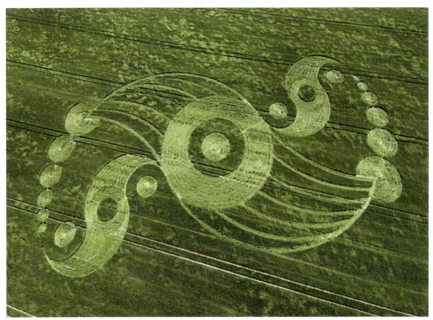

United Kingdom, Wiltshire, Windmill Hill, nr. Avebury
25 May, 2009

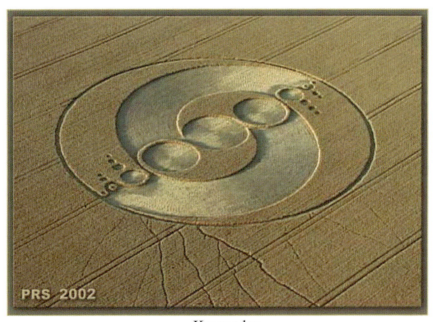

Krasnodar

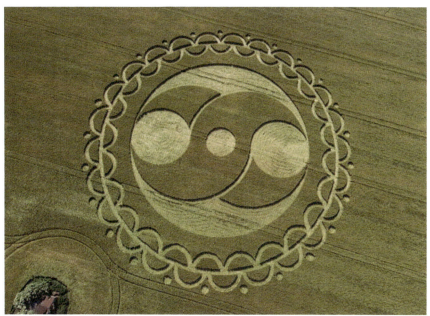

June 20, 2008, Furze Knoll, Wiltshire, UK

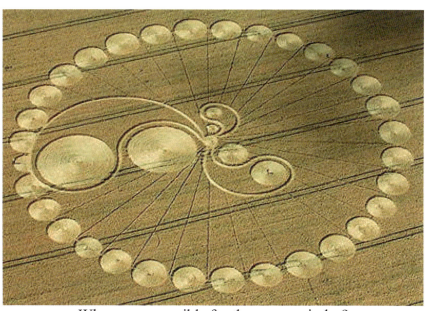

Who are responsible for those crop circles?

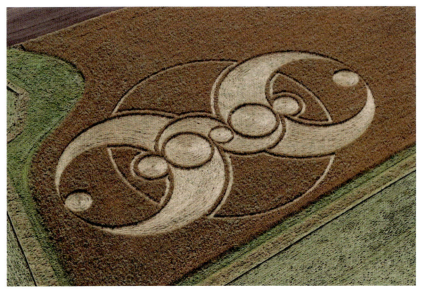

What do they want to tell us in those circles?

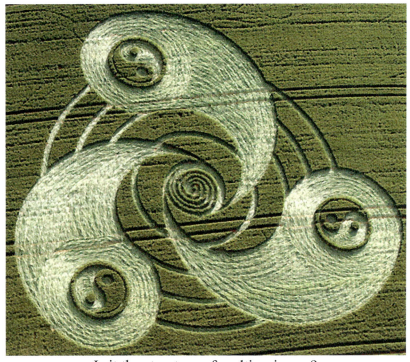

Is it the structure of multi-universe?

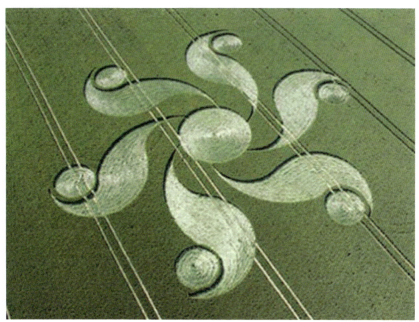

Why there are so many circles in Taiji shape?

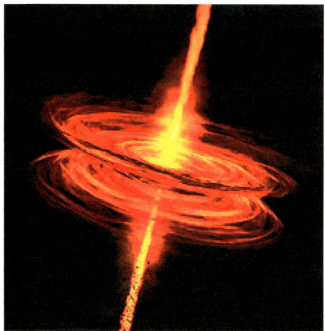

Dao that can be described is not universal and eternal Dao

# 3 HU TU IS THE NUMEROLOGY MODEL OF TAIJI

Dated back to 6500 and 10,000 years ago, there were 2 diagrams of the stars that appeared in central China. One is called He Tu, (Yellow) River Diagram, one is called Luo Shu, Luo (river) Diagram. The 2 diagrams are more than a map of stars, but rather are a cosmological model. In the 2 diagrams, dots were used as numbers because there were no characters at that time. Based on those 2 diagrams, the first emperor in Chinese history, created Bagua, eight trigrams. This is considered the beginning of Chinese culture.

He Tu is the origin of Five Elements theory. Before He Tu, it is estimated that Chinese medicine had been used for 600,000 years or so. However, until He Tu came to China, Chinese medicine had no system.

If we say Chinese medicine is very complicated, yes, it is.
If we say Chinese medicine is very simple, yes, it is.
All is just in a He Tu diagram.

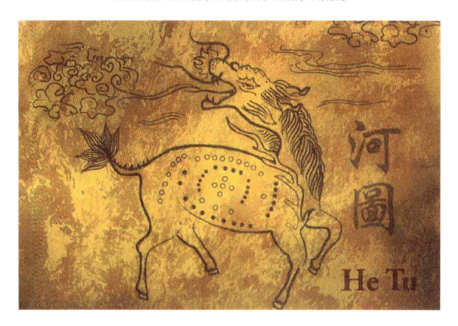

According to legend, the He Tu was derived from the sighting of a unique creature, during the era of the sage Fu Xi in China. The dragon-headed horse with carp-like scales was spotted at the Yellow River. Its body contained unique and strange markings which were noted by the sages and then studied in depth. After much detailed study of the markings, the sages concluded that the markings on the horse could be arranged into a model of dots. This model was named the He Tu or River Map.

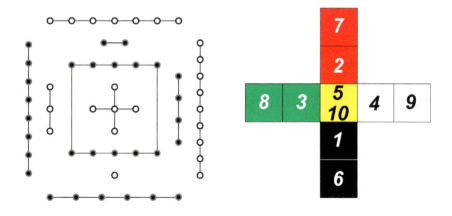

He Tu

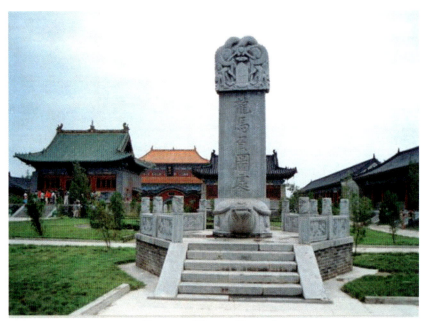

Dragon Horse Temple

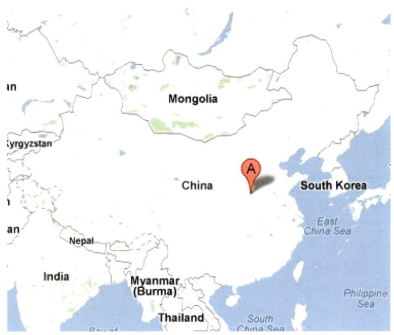

Location of the Dragon Horse Temple

In the eyes of the ancient Chinese people, the five major stars (planets) in the solar system appeared on different directions of the sky. This was recorded on a diagram of dots. Now we can see them on He Tu.

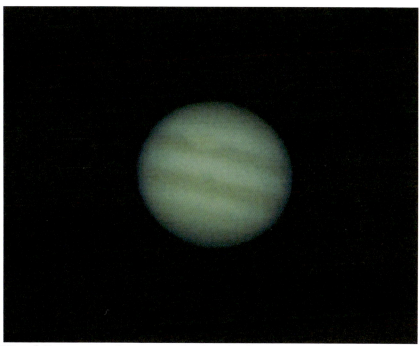

Wood Star, green, known as Jupiter in the east, on the dates with 3 and 8 in Chinese calendar, e.g. 3, 8; 13, 18; 23, 28, appears on the eastern sky, represents the left side of the He Tu diagram.

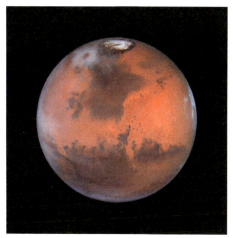

Fire Star, red, known as Mars in the south, on the dates with 2and 7 in Chinese calendar, e.g. 2, 7; 12, 17; 22, 27, appears on the southern sky, represents the top of He Tu diagram.

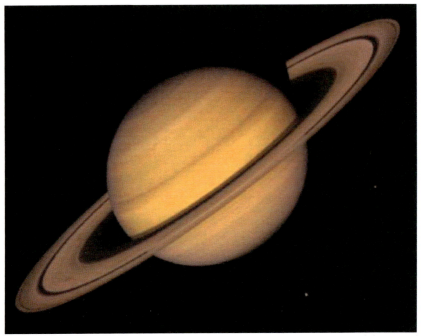

Earth Star, yellow, known as Saturn above, on the dates with 5 and 10 in Chinese calendar, e.g. 5, 10; 15, 20; 25, 30 appears directly on the sky above, represents the middle of He Tu diagram.

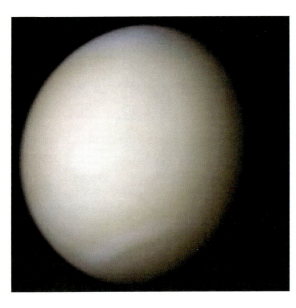

Metal Star, white, known as Venus in the west, on the dates with 4 and 9 in Chinese calendar, e.g. 4, 9; 14, 19; 24, 29 appears on the western sky, represents the right of side of the He Tu diagram.

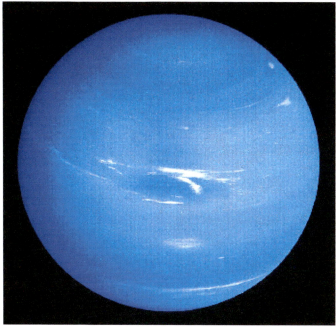

Water Star, blue, known as Mercury in the north, on the dates with 1 and 6 in Chinese calendar, e.g. 1, 6; 11, 16; 21, 26 appears on the northern sky, represents the bottom of He Tu diagram.

Combined with the theory of Yin and Yang, the He Tu serves as the primary system of Chinese medicine since its inception. Odd numbers are Yang numbers, even numbers are Yin numbers. Five Elements came from the directions of East/Left/Green/Wood, West/Right/White/Metal, South/Top/Red/Fire, North/Bottom/Blue/Water and Middle/Yellow/Earth.

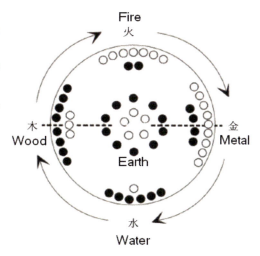

Yang Qi ascends on the left and descends on the right; fully activated on the top and stored in the bottom.

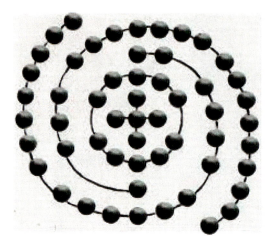

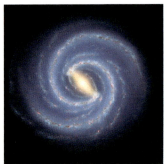

He Tu in Nebula Shape

天地之气，合而为一

Qi from heaven and the Earth,
when in intercourse they are one

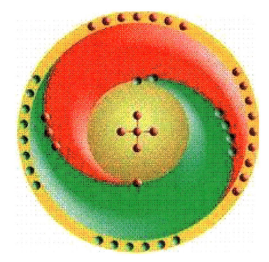

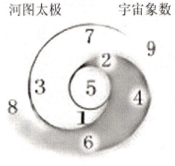

Numerology in He Tu

分为阴阳

When separated into two forms,
they are Yin and Yang

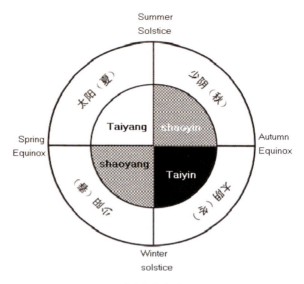

判为四时

When in time pattern, they are four seasons

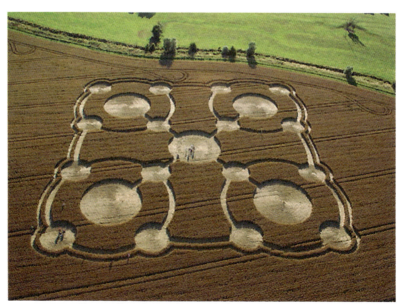

Sprouting in spring, Thriving in summer
Harvesting in autumn, Storing in winter

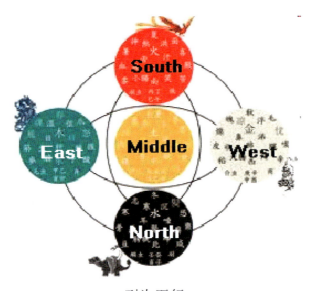

列为五行
When in direction pattern, they are Five Elements in space model

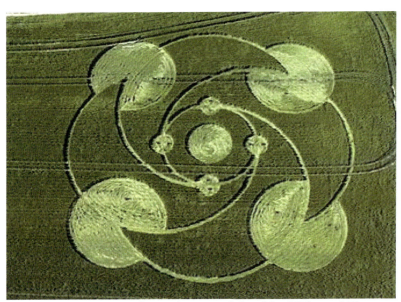

Five elements are the pathways of the Qi of Yin and Yang

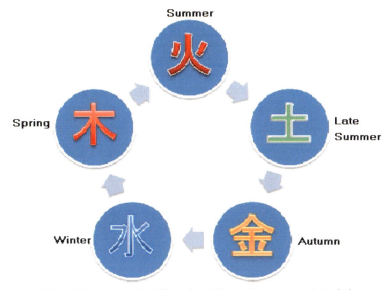

Five Elements in Circular Time Sequence Model

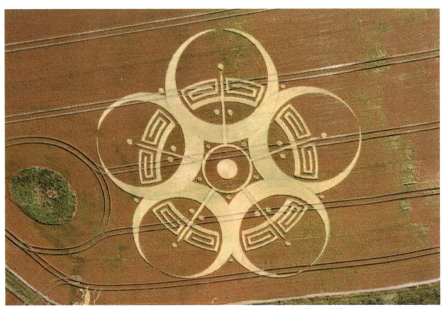

The Five Stars Circulate Qi in Forms of Five Elements

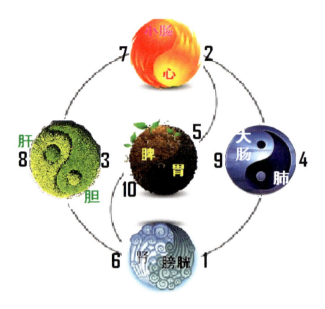

He Tu – The System of Chinese Medicine

East:       8, Wood-Yin, Liver      3, Wood-Yang, Gallbladder
South:     2, Fire-Yin, Heart       7, Fire-Yang, Small Intestine
Middle:   10, Earth-Yin, Spleen 5, Earth-Yang, Stomach
West:      4, Metal-Yin, Lung      9, Metal Yang, Large Intestine
North:     6, Water-Yin, Kidney 1, Water-Yang, Bladder

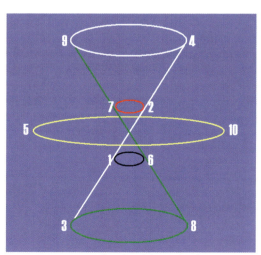

He Tu in double spiral

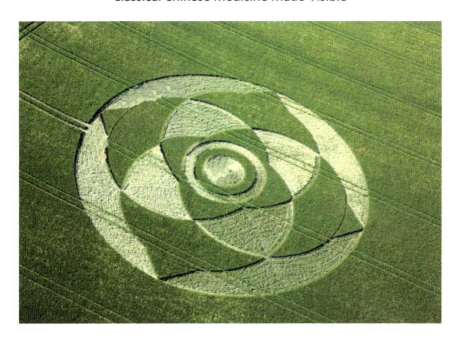

Five elements material is on the Earth, their Qi is over the sky

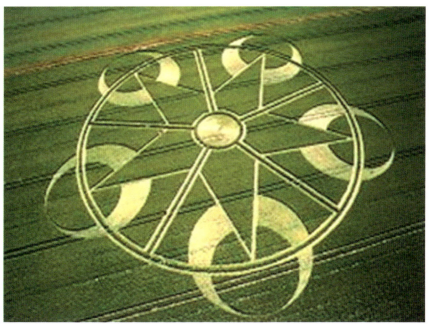

Since the universe was created
'the Fives' have been circulating over the sky

# 4 LUO SHU, MAP OF STARS

Luo Shu, similar to He Tu, is also the numerologic model of Taiji.

Luo Shu was derived from big dipper and north star system. The North Star was called the emperor, the big dipper was the carrier that takes the emperor going around the heaven. Compared to He Tu which was derived from the planets of the solar system.

Luo Shu focuses on Yin and Yang. He Tu focuses on Five Elements.

The universal principles are reflected in these two cosmological models. There is no limit to the applications of these principles, they can be applied to the sky, the Earth and the human body.

Being applied to the sky, it is astrology and calendar; being applied to the Earth, it is Feng Shui; being applied to the human body, it is Chinese medicine.

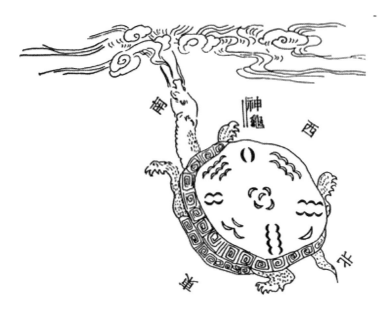

Chinese legends concerning the pre-historic Emperor Yu tell of the Luo Shu, often in connection with the He Tu and 8 trigrams. In ancient China there was a great flood: the people offered sacrifices to the god of one of the flooding rivers, the Luo river , to try to calm his anger. A magical turtle emerged from the water with the curious and decidedly unnatural Lo Shu pattern on its shell: circular dots giving binary representations of the integers one through nine are arranged in a three-by-three grid.

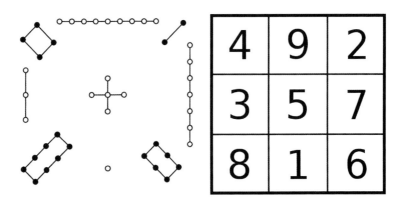

Luo Shu

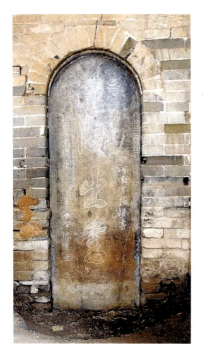

Ancient Monument of Luo Shu

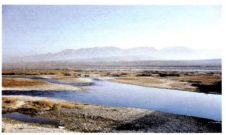

Luo River

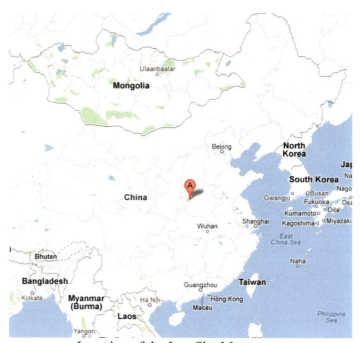

Location of the Luo Shu Monument

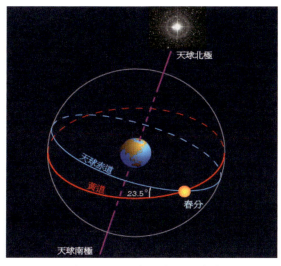

The sky is like a cover, the north star (Polaris) is the central axis. This axis also represents the concept and the importance of the center or the middle. Its property is half Yin and half Yang, but has no concept of time or direction. It may be infinitely small, or it may be all encompassing. It is the origin from which the other four phenomena revolve.

In the five elements, the Earth is in the middle. It is compatible to others, creates others and is superior to others. In this sense, Polaris was considered the emperor of the stars.

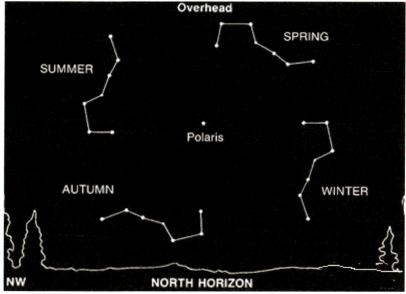

The emperor goes around the heaven with his carrier. Four seasons are shown by the handle of the dipper. Does this look like a huge clock?

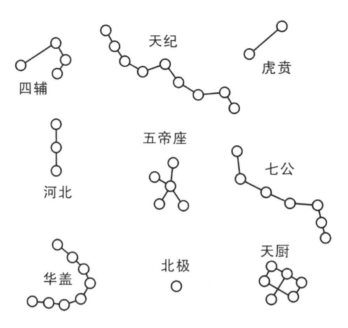

Map of the Nine Constellations

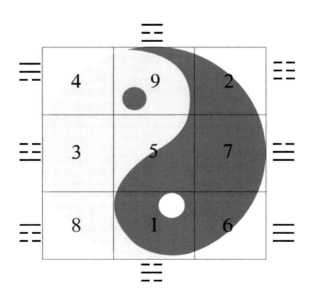

Nine Halls

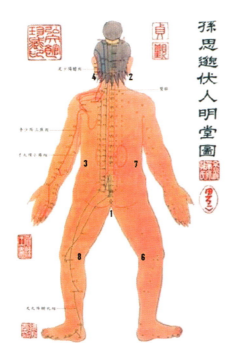

Top nine bottom one
Left three right seven
Two and four are shoulders
Six and eight are the feet
five in the middle

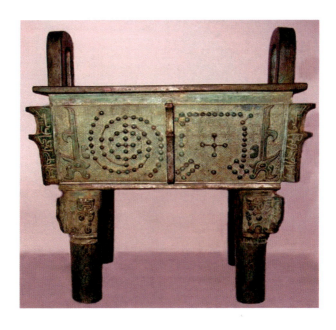

He Tu and Luo Shu are the Origin of Chinese Culture

# 5 CLASSICAL CHINESE MEDICINE:
# SELF-CONSISTENT SYSTEM

"Medicine started from Emperor Fuxi, developed by Emperor Shennong and Huangdi, has been spreading over thousands of years and will last forever. It based on Dao and follows the nature" (Liu, Wansu, 1110~1200 ).

Foundation of Classical Chinese Medicine is formed by two parts:

1. Theory: three classics in the early ancient times, 上古三坟 （3000 BC-21Century BC)

| | |
|---|---|
| Fuxi Bagua | 伏羲八卦 |
| Shennong's Materia Medica | 神农本草经 |
| Yellow Emperor's Inner Canon | 黄帝内经 |

2. Technique: Three Preferred Classics, "do not take treatment from doctors who havn't read the three classics", 医不三世，不服其药

| | |
|---|---|
| Huangdi's Acupuncture | 灵枢 |
| Shennong's Materia Medica | 神农本草经 |
| Su-nyu's Pulse Diagnosis | 素女脉诀 |

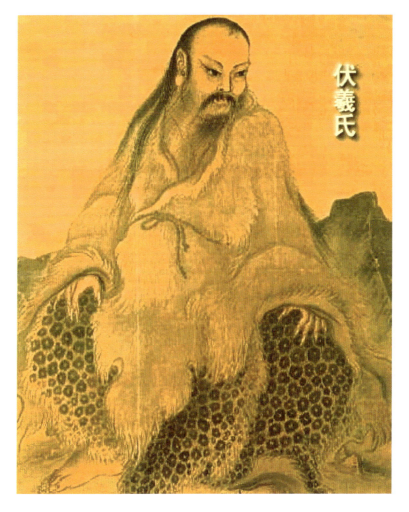

Fuxi, Created Nine Needles and Bagua

Fu Xi was the originator of the Yi Jing, whose work is attributed to his reading of the He Tu and Luo Shu. According to this tradition, Fu Xi had drawn the first stroke of the trigrams which started the Chinese culture. Fu Xi also made the arrangement of the trigrams revealed to him supernaturally. This arrangement precedes the compilation of the Yi Jing during the Zhou dynasty. Yi Jing is the philosophy of Classical Chinese Medicine.

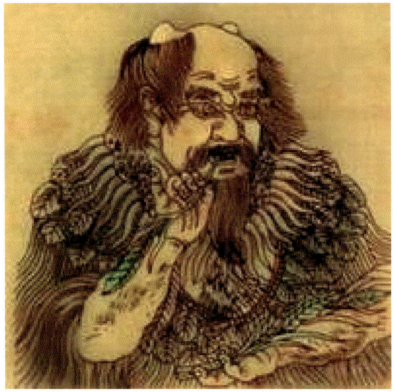

Shennong, tasted herbs and created Mountain Yi

Prior to the legend of Shennong, people were sickly, wanting, starved and diseased; but he then taught them agriculture, which he himself had researched, eating hundreds of plants — and even consuming seventy poisons in one day. Shennong also created in the book Mountain Yi.

The Shennong's Materia Medica is a book on agriculture and medicinal plants, attributed to Shennong. Researcher suggests that it is a compilation of oral traditions, written between about 300 BCE and 200 CE.

There is a school in Classical Chinese Medicine known as Classical Formula School. Shennong is the father of this school. Yin Yi, who began to work as a cook for the emperor, later became a minister, wrote a book named Tang Ye Jing (汤液经，Decoction Classics). Unfortunately, Tang Ye Jing went missing, but luckily enough some of it's formula were inherited and retained in Shang Han Lun. The Tang Ye Jing pentagonic diagram was retained in a book "Fu Xing Jue". It summarized the connection between the functions and bodies, rules to form formula according to the major category of syndromes.

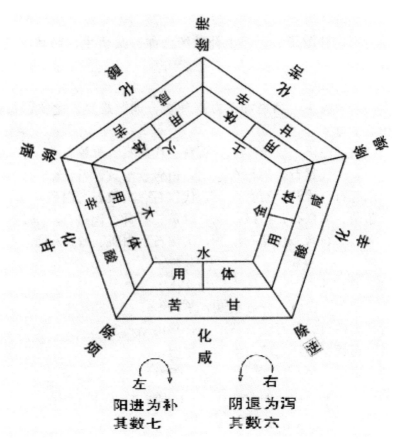

"This is diagram of rules of Tang Ye Jing with all importance in it. Learners who understand this complete all the study of medicine".

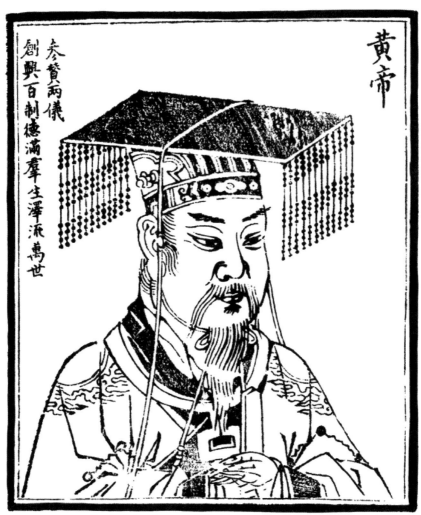

Huangdi, finished Inner Cannon and created Earth Yi

Yellow Emperor's Inner Canon is composed of two texts each of eighty-one chapters or treatises in a question-and-answer format between the mythical Huangdi (Yellow Emperor) and six of his equally legendary ministers. This book is still the foundation of Chinese medicine which developed into a school known as Medical Classics School.

All the Three Sovereigns, Fuxi, Shennong and Huangdi contributed to both Yi Jing and medicine.

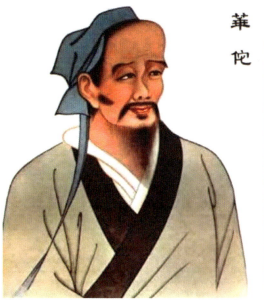

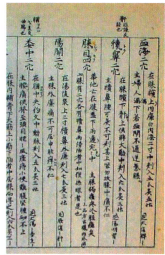

Huatuo, the top acupuncturist (145-208 DC), the author of "Qing Nang Shu" (Black Bag Book), the book was missing.

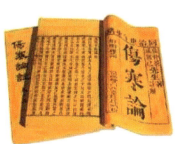

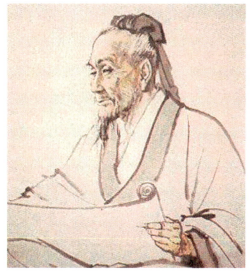

Zhang, Zhongjing, the top herbalist, 150-219 DC, the author of "Shang Han Lun"

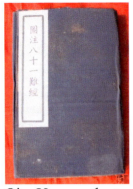

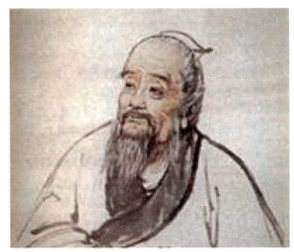

Qin, Yueren, the top pulse specialist (407-310 BC), the author of "On Eighty One Difficult Questions"

The scope of Classical Chinese Medicine can be summarized by the "Four Great Classics";
Yellow Emperor's Inner Canon, covers the basic theory and acupuncture;
Shennong's Materia Medica, covers the herbology;
On Eighty One Difficult Questions, covers pulse diagnosis;
Shang Han Lun, covers classical formula in six stage diagnostic system.

**Classical Chinese Medicine** is a special medical system based on ancient astrology. It uses Yi Jing as a philosophical foundation, and is characterized by imagery and numerological thinking. It treats illness primarily by regulating Qi and it uses pulse as an essential part of the diagnosis. This Medicine reached its pinnacle during the Han and Tang dynasties. It presents a systemic medicine based on experience, and is governed by practices derived from the observation of stable phenomena in nature. These practices are, in turn, described by means of axioms in its self-consistent theories, logical deductions, and numerological calculations.

During the process of human evolution, there are usually three ways to discover truth: religion, philosophy, and science. Science is the most precise method; religion is the most cursory, while the philosophical approaches fall in the middle as the most balanced. In the past 500 years, we humans have learned that the scientific method provides an effective model to understand the natural realm, so we also apply the same approach to explore the fields of thinking and spirituality. Eventually, we learned to apply the scientific approach to all unchartered territory, from astronomy to thinking, spirituality, neurology, and consciousness. However, when scientists face difficulties such as when they attempt to understand and explicate new areas like quantum mechanics, in addition to the methods of the natural science, human beings can only draw on logical thinking and philosophical speculation to reach the conclusions they seek.

As a holistic modality, Chinese Medicine had no other choice but to use a combination of authentication and speculation to understand the heavens, the earth, and human beings during its advent and developing period. In the macro world, human cognition and the acquisition of knowledge of the truth require a high degree of philosophical reflection. This is what the ancient Greek philosopher, Aristotle, meant by "inductive logic". It was this approach that was used to derive one phenomenon from another, to go from individuals to groups, and to shift from the special material nature to the universal material nature. This is the reason why Chinese Medicine adopted analog as a research method. It started with axioms and supposition and, unless it found counter examples, it firmly believed that those starting points were not only correct but, could also provide the basis to apply judgments based on general principles to specific areas. Under this system, the principle of the micro-world knowledge to the test of truth is no longer a measurement or a direct proof. Its objective becomes to predict results in which no counter-examples exist. If the results are consistent and there are no counter-examples, the self-consistent system can be established with relative success.

"Self-consistency is a system that is consistent with one's self or with itself. It is not self-contradictory, nor a deviation from the ordinary standard by which the conduct is guided. Logically it is consistent throughout; with each component in harmony with the rest."

"An axiom, or postulate, is a premise or starting point for reasoning. As classically conceived, an axiom is a premise as evident as to be accepted as true without controversy. An axiom can be any mathematical statement that serves as a starting point from which other statements can be logically derived. Within the system they define, axioms (unless redundant) cannot be derived by principles of deduction, nor are they demonstrable by mathematical proofs simply because they are starting points. There is nothing else from which they logically follow otherwise they would be classified as theorems. However, an axiom in one system can become be a theorem in another, and vice versa."

Axioms can build a complete and "no contradiction" system to meet the consistency of a theoretical system. Almost all of the areas of mathematics and even some scientific fields outside of mathematics draw on the axiomatic system to construct their theories. Einstein's theory of relativity and Hawking's theories of time and space are based on such understandings.

Here are some examples of axioms in Chinese Medicine:

1, All that is in the process of being created or in movement in the universe needs energy (known as primordial Qi or Taiji).

2. There are day and night in every day (known as Yin and Yang).

3. There are four seasons in a year (known as four phenomena).

4. The earth orientation is divided into east, west, south, north, and middle (known as five elements).

5. Although everything in the world has relevance, some components are stronger, and some are weaker (known as analog method).

6 The motion of celestial bodies affects the earth (known as the earth responds to the sky).

7. Human beings are part of the universe (known as human

responds to the heaven).

8. All the creatures in the world have their birth and death (known as the birth, growth, transformation, resizing, and storage).

9. All the movements of the universe are in endless circles (known as circular motion and Zi Wu circulation).

Axioms are set up for the convenience of study, under certain circumstances based on specific standards. it is possible to carry out deeper research. This standard is the axiom. The axioms are independent and do not need to be proven. They become the habitual usage or a stable theoretical system in which it is inconvenient to make changes. They can also be so general that it becomes impossible to use them in the existing theory to develop a general height (such as $1 + 1 = 2$). In this sense, the classics of Chinese Medicine can become the works on axioms for the healing modality. Classics cannot be changed and can only serve as foundations for further interpretations.

As a self-consistent system, Classic Chinese Medicine must have a stable ideological model to follow. This ideological model is Yi Jing, the philosophical foundation of Chinese Medicine. It is only within this stability, that one can use the term "classic". In this self-consistent system, any answer to the basic questions of Classical Chinese Medicine must conform to this model. Otherwise, Classical Chinese Medicine will no longer form a self-consistent system. Efforts to seek answers from outside the system will deviate from the self-consistent character of Chinese Medicine. Then the result cannot be considered to be Classic Chinese Medicine any longer. The resulting modality can only be called "modern" Chinese Medicine. The term "Modern" implies change because nothing can remain "modern" forever. It is of great necessity and importance for Yi Jing to remain the philosophical foundation of all Classical Chinese Medicine.

A self-consistent system is independent. It does not need to be proven or to be supported by other systems. The argument about whether Chinese Medicine is scientific should be discontinued.

First, let's take a look of the definition of science:

1, Science on broad sense: "**Science** (from Latin *scientia*, meaning 'knowledge') is a systematic enterprise that builds and organizes knowledge in the form of testable explanations and predictions about the universe. In an older and closely related meaning, "science" also refers to a body of knowledge itself, of the type that can be rationally explained and reliably applied. Since classical antiquity, science as a type of knowledge has been closely linked to philosophy. In the early modern period, the words 'science' and 'philosophy' were sometimes used interchangeably. By the 17th century, natural philosophy (which is today called 'natural science') was considered a separate branch of philosophy. However, 'science' continued to be used in a broad sense denoting reliable knowledge about a topic, in the same way it is still used in modern terms such as in library science or political science.

2, Science on narrow sense: "In modern use, 'science' more often refers to a way of pursuing knowledge, not only the knowledge itself. It is often treated as synonymous with 'natural and physical science', and thus restricted to those branches of study that relate to the phenomena of the material universe and its laws, sometimes with implied exclusion of pure mathematics. This is now the dominant sense in ordinary use. This is the narrower sense of 'science'. Recently, it has become more common to refer to natural philosophy as 'natural science'. Over the course of the 19th century, the word 'science' became increasingly associated with the scientific method, a disciplined way to study the natural world This definition of science is frequently applied to academic disciplines such as physics, chemistry, geology, and biology. "

So there are two kinds of definitions of sciences: one broad and one narrow. It is the narrow classification that has generated the controversy about whether Chinese Medicine is scientific or not. By the broad definition, there is no doubt that Chinese Medicine is scientific; by the narrow one, it may not be. It is neither realistic nor necessary to insist that Chinese Medicine must meet the standards of the narrow definition of science since, as a healing system, it predates the concept of science by a few thousand years.

Secondly, science is not necessarily synonymous with the truth, if by truth we mean the world as it is. Knowledge is the level of awareness of the world as it is. Science is only one of the paths toward that truth. It is, by no means, the only path. If we take science as being the whole and only truth, then much of what we accept as science today can fall into the realm of superstition. As Einstein and Hawking illustrate, we cannot experience everything that is scientific through our physical senses.

Natural phenomena can be divided into two types: 1) natural phenomena within the range of ordinary physical experience; 2) natural phenomena outside the range of ordinary physical experience. Modern science and its objectives are defined within the ordinary physical experience of sound, sight, touch, taste, smell, pressure, and pain. In addition to the four diagnoses of observing, smelling, asking and touching in the range of ordinary physical experience, Chinese Medicine also acknowledges the existence of "meridians", "Qi", and "spirit," all of which fall outside the ordinary physical experience. In fact, Chinese Medicine maintains that there is no supernatural phenomenon. There are only natural phenomena. It is only because of the limitations of modern science and technology that the so-called supernatural phenomena exist.

"Usual phenomena" which can be observed, are only statistically significant for a majority of people, most of the time, in most of the cases, for most possibilities. The rest belong to the "unusual phenomena". In this sense, the connection between Chinese Medicine and the natural world comes closer to the truth than does the link between the world and modern medicine.

Thirdly, in the nineteenth century, the gunboats of the Western countries forcibly opened the doors to China. After continuous failures as a consequence of the huge gap between their level of science and technology and that of Europe, the Qing Dynasty's attitude towards to the West was permanently altered. It shifted from contempt to being forced to learn. During the Opium Wars, China not only suffered defeat on the battlefield, but was also forced to compromise its identity. This experience was completely different from those of its previous foreign invasions. In the past, despite the defeats, Chinese people remained confident that their own civilization was indisputably superior to that of their opponents. It can be said that, in the past five thousand years of history, China had not encountered a civilization it considered superior to itself. But this time, the Chinese people's attitude towards the West changed dramatically. It shifted from the exclusion of the past to the gradual acceptance of "total Westernization". Because in the first Sino-Japanese war China was defeated by a small country like Japan, it was thrown into turmoil of disgrace and self-denial.

This change has been reflected in all aspects of Chinese Medicine.

Objectively, it forced Classic Chinese Medicine to change into modern Western science. The result of this change is that Classic Chinese medicine has been severely emasculated. As a consequence of this, in the country of its origin,

Chinese Medicine has been subjected to unprecedented levels of ridiculous embarrassment. Since then, whether Chinese medicine treatments are right or wrong have had to be determined by Western medicinal standards. This unusual situation, in which the efficacy of one discipline must be judged by the standards of a different one, I am afraid, is extremely rare in the history of science. In order to survive, Chinese Medicine has had to under go "modernization." This is a bit like having to cut the feet to fit shoes. The result has led us to question whether Classic Chinese Medicine is of sufficient value to warrant its existence. The independent complete system of classic Chinese Medicine has almost become a well guarded secret.

In the past half century, the philosophy of Classical Chinese

Medicine has been taken away and it has been replaced by the political philosophy of materialist dialectics. Statistics show that the doctors of the Han (206bc-220ce) and Tang (618-906ce) Dynasties, who understood the Yi Jing accounted for 85%of the practitioners. During the Ming Dynasty (1368-1644ce), this figure dropped to only 12%. Sadly, if we were to do the same research today, the results would likely be even more disappointing. What were the requirements in Inner Cannon for Chinese medicine doctors? The "Nei Jing" declared the following: "To be a doctor, one must know the heaven above, the earth below and the human in the middle." Now this dictum has become little more than empty, meaningless talk.

To alter the classics is to ignore their origin. This had already happened to Classical Chinese medicine in ancient times. However, compared to those who are trying to "modernize" Chinese medicine today, the betrayers in the old times are really dwarfed. The hidden objective of the modernization of Chinese Medicine is to explain it with the existing human knowledge rather than to transform it drawing on the beautiful words of "science" in the narrow sense. The principles of Traditional Chinese Medicine were derived from the universe close to "Dao," or the Source. Compared to those in modern medicine, concepts in Chinese Medicine are much broader. If Chinese and Western medicine must be unified successfully and fairly, then the narrow concepts must follow the broad ones and not vice versa.

# Chronology of Classical Chinese Medicine

| Date | Dynasty | Subdivision | Capital |
|------|---------|-------------|---------|
| ca. 1600-1050 BC | Shang （商） | | Near present-day Zhengzhou and Anyang |
| ca. 1046-771 BC | Zhou （周） | Western Zhou | Hao (near present-day Xi'an) |
| ca. 771-475 BC | | Spring and Autumn Period * | Luoyang (in present-day Henan) |
| ca. 475-221 BC | | Warring States Period * | |
| 206 BC-9 AD** | Han （汉） | Western Han | Chang'an (present-day Xi'an) |
| 25-220 AD | | Eastern Han | Luoyang |
| 220-265 AD | 6 Dynasties Period | 3 Kingdoms Period | No Unified Capital |
| 265-420 AD | | Jin (晉) Dynasty | Luoyang, then Jiankang (Nanjing) |
| 386-589 AD | | Northern and Southern Dynasties Period | No Unified Capital (several dynasties at Jiankang) |
| 581-618 AD | Sui (隋) | | Daxing (Chang'an) |
| 618-906 AD | Tang （唐） | | Chang'an, then Luoyang |

# 6 EIGHT TRIGRAMS

无极生有极、有极是太极
太极生两仪、即阴阳
两仪生四象、即少阴、太阴、少阳、太阳
四象演八卦、八八六十四卦

Wuji which is without polarity, produces polarity which is the Taiji.
Taiji produces two forms, which are yin and yang.
The two forms produce four phenomena, named Lesser Yin, Greater Yin (Tai Yin also means the moon), Lesser Yang, Greater Yang (Tai Yang also means the Sun).
The four phenomena divide into the eight trigrams (Bagua), and then eight times eight are the sixty-four hexagrams.

Taiji is a circle, it exists everywhere and is larger then the largest and smaller then the smallest. Before Taiji was formed, it was like a black hole containing limitless potential, and was known as Wuji. As it initially exists as a point of singularity, and from the perspective of its circle alone, the Taiji represents primordial Qi; from the perspective of the duality it contains, it is Yin and Yang; Taiji as five, it is Five Elements; Taiji as eight, it is Eight Trigrams. Taiji can then be divided into 64, and like the 64 hexagrams are the 64 codes of the universe.

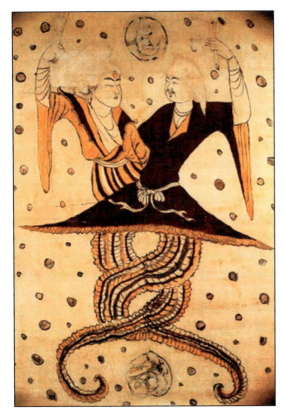

At Fuxi's time, there were no characters. Fuxi had to find a simple way to share his idea. The way he found was the combination of 2 kinds of lines, a straight line and a broken line which were called Yao. The straight line is Yang Yao, the broken line is Yin Yao.

Fuxi and his wife Nyuwa in legend. Their tales formed into double spiral.

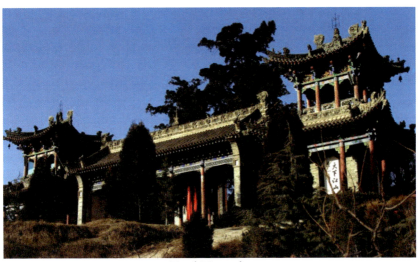

Fuxi Temple

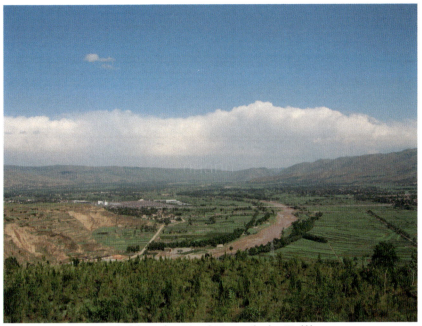

Field under Fuxi Temple in Taiji

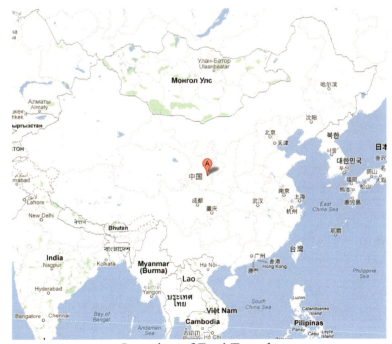

Location of Fuxi Temple

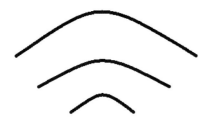

If we need to draw the continuous sky, are the 3 lines like this, the simple and best way?
This is Qian, the sky.

If we draw the Earth, what it should look like? The Earth is not continuous, so broken lines were used.
This is Kun, the Earth.

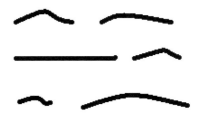

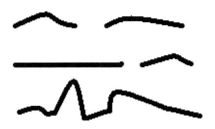

What if the lowest layer under the Earth moves? That is the Earthquake.
This is Zhen, the thunder.

What moves in the middle part of the Earth? It must be water.
This is Kan, the water

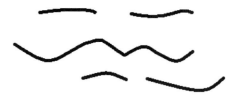

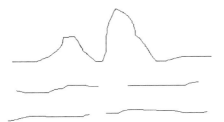

What if the surface of the Earth moves? It forms mountains.
This is Gen, the mountains.

What moves in the lowest layer of the sky and on the surface of the Earth? It is the wind. This is Xun, the wind.

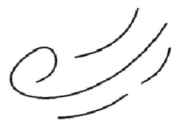

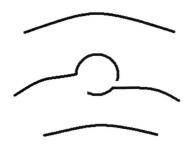

What is the most attractive object moves in the middle part of the sky? Sun. This is Li, the Sun.

What is there in the top of the sky? Black hole, the opening to connect the other universe.
This is Dui, the lake which is also the opening on the Earth.

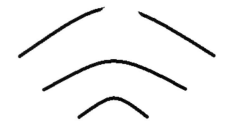

Taiji creates two forms: Yin and Yang

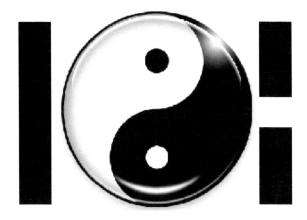

Two Forms create four phenomena:
Tai Yin, Tai Yang, Shao Yin, Shao Yang

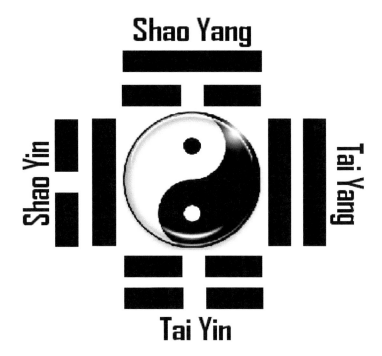

Four phenomena create eight trigrams

1 ䷀ 乾 QIÁN　天 HEAVEN/SKY
2 ䷹ 兑 DUÌ　泽 LAKE/MARSH
3 ䷝ 离 LÍ　火 FIRE
4 ䷲ 震 ZHÈN　雷 THUNDER
5 ䷸ 巽 XÙN　风 WIND
6 ䷜ 坎 KǍN　水 WATER
7 ䷳ 艮 GÈN　山 MOUNTAIN
8 ䷁ 坤 KŪN　地 EARTH

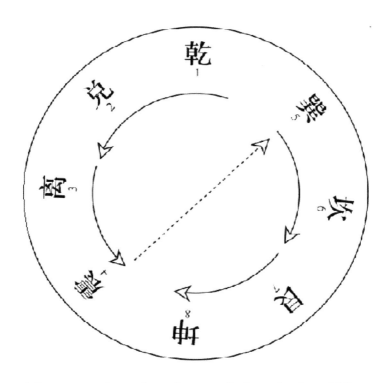

The pre-natal numbers form an S shape in the middle.

道生一，一生二，二生三，三生万物
Dao creates one, one creates two
two creates three, three creates all

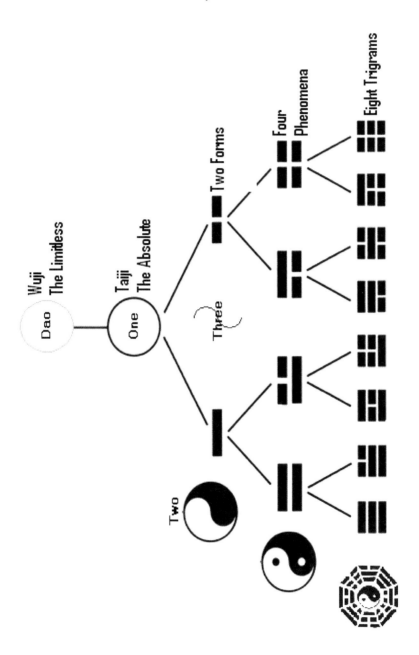

# PRE-NATAL BAGUA

| 卦名 Name | 自然 Nature | 季节 Season | 性情 Personality | 象族 Family | 方位 Direction | 意畫 Meaning |
|---|---|---|---|---|---|---|
| 乾 Qián | 天 Sky (Heaven) | Summer | Creative | 父 Father | 南 South | Expansive energy, the sky. For further information. |
| 巽 Xùn | 風 Wind | Summer | Gentle | 長女 Eldest Daughter | 西南 Southwest | Gentle penetration, flexibility. |
| 坎 Kǎn | 水 Water | Autumn | Abysmal | 中男 Middle Son | 西 West | Danger, rapid rivers, the abyss, the moon. |
| 艮 Gèn | 山 Mountain | Autumn | Still | 少男 Youngest Son | 西北 North-west | Stillness, immovability. |
| 坤 Kūn | 地 Earth | Winter | Receptive | 母 Mother | 北 North | Receptive energy, that which yields. For further information. |
| 震 Zhèn | 雷 Thunder | Winter | Arousing | 長男 Eldest Son | 東北 North-east | Excitation, revolution, division. |
| 離 Lí | 火 Fire | Spring | Clinging | 中女 Middle Daughter | 東 East | Rapid movement, radiance, the sun. |
| 兌 Duì | 澤 Lake | Spring | Joyous | 少女 Youngest Daughter | 東南 Southeast | Joy, satisfaction, stagnation. |

How Fuxi draw the Bagua based on He Tu and Luo Shu? Let's try to repeat this process.

Step 1: Taiji creates Bagua. Get the numbers for 4 signs and 8 trigrams, the numbers for each trigrams are pre-natal Bagua numbers;

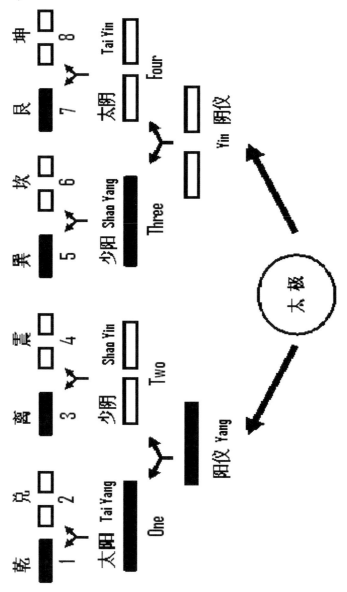

Step 2: Put the four signs into He Tu according to their numbers;

Step 3: Put the trigrams under the four signs into He Tu and get their numbers from He Tu;

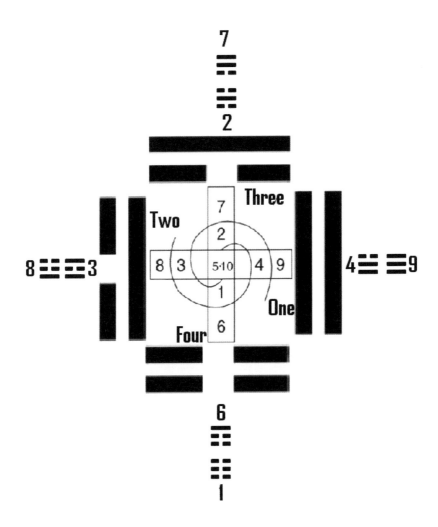

Step 4. Now the numbers in the diagram above are the numbers for Luo Shu.

| 8 | 7 | 6 | 5 | 4 | 3 | 2 | 1 |
|---|---|---|---|---|---|---|---|
| 地 | 山 | 水 | 風 | 雷 | 火 | 澤 | 天 |
| ☷ | ☶ | ☵ | ☴ | ☳ | ☲ | ☱ | ☰ |
| 1 | 6 | 7 | 2 | 8 | 3 | 4 | 9 |

5

Step 5. Arrange the trigrams into Luo Shu according to the numbers in the above chart;

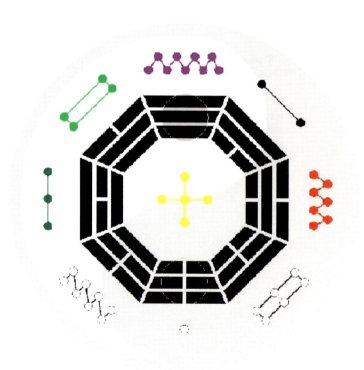

Now we got the Fuxi Bagua or Pre-natal Bagua.

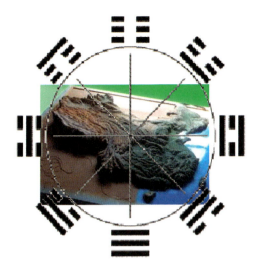

Heaven and the Earth
are located;
Air circulates among
mountains and lakes;
Wind swipes the land
with Thunder;
The Sun (fire) and the
moon (water) are
spinning over the sky
alternatively.
What an alive landscape
of China.

The creator is the pre-natal, the being created is post-natal.
Wuji (limitless potential), mother of Taiji, is considered pre-natal,
Taiji, being created by Wuji, is considered post-natal;
Taiji as one Qi, which divided into Yin and Yang, is prenatal. Yin
and Yang, being created by one Qi, is considered post-natal;
Pre-natal Qi is without shape, sound or smell, post-natal beings are
with forms, signs and structure;
Compared to Five Elements, Yin and Yang are pre-natal.
Compared to Yin and Yang, Five Elements are post-natal.

Pre-natal Bagua is the
structure of Yi. It reflects
the nature, so the sky is on
the top and the Earth is on
the bottom. Taiji is divided
into left and right by Qian-
Kun line

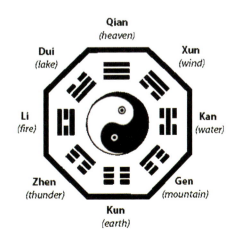

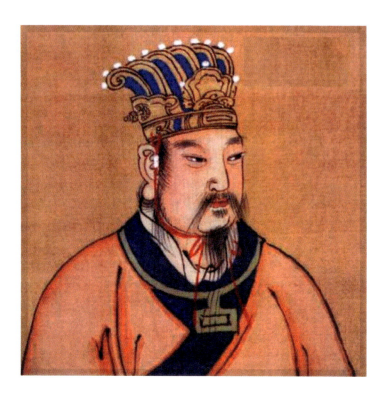

King Wen of Zhou (1152 – 1056 BC) set up a kingdom known as Zhou dynasty. His devotion to Yi is called Zhou Yi.

Based on the pre-natal Bagua, King Wen drew the post-natal Bagua to fit the Five Element model.
The post-natal Bagua is the function of Yi. It reflects weather, so the fire is on the south and the water is on the north. Taiji is divided into up and down by Zhen-Dui line.

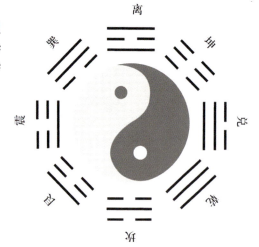

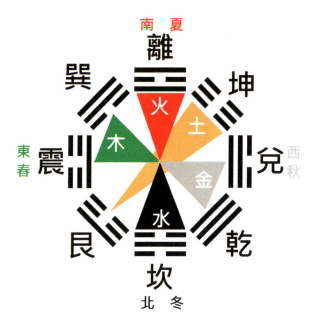

The post-natal Bagua gains the property of Five Elements

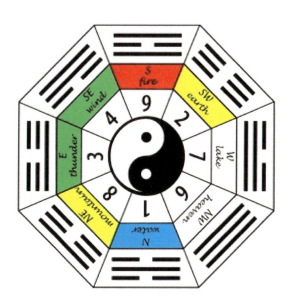

The post-natal Bagua gets its numbers from Luo Shu

# 7 SIXTY FOUR HEXAGRAMS
# THE CODES OF THE UNIVERSE

King Wen of Zhou (1152 – 1056 BC) was king of Zhou during the late Shang dynasty in ancient China. Although it was his son Wu who conquered the Shang following the Battle of Muye, King Wen was honored as the founder of the Zhou dynasty. Some consider him the first epic hero of Chinese history.

King Wen doubled the trigrams got 64 hexagrams (Gua, symble). According to the combinations and connections of the 2 upper and lower trigrams, locations of Yin or Yang Yao, King Wen named each Gua, wrote text for each Gua and made the sequences of 64 hexagrams. Wu continued his work, wrote text for each of 384 yao.

"立天之道曰阴阳，立地之道曰柔刚，立人之道曰仁义，兼三才而两之，故六画而成卦"。 "Dao of the heaven is Yin and Yang; Dao of the Earth is softness and hardness; the Dao of human is kindness and justice. Those are the three vitals with two yao in each vital go to six yao forming hexagram".

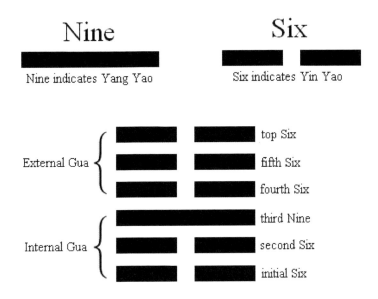

中，zhong, means middle which is favorable position of the external or internal Gua.

正，zheng, means match that initial, 3, 5 are Yang position; 2, 4, top are Yin position. It is favorable Zheng for Yang yao on Yang position and Yin yao on Yin position.

承，cheng, means support that Yang yao is supported by one or more Yin yao directly under it.

乘，also pronounced cheng, means Yang yao is suppressed by one or more Yin yao above it.

比，bi, means adjacent that 2 yao locate one after the other. Good bi is to make Yin and Yang together.

应，ying, means response that refers to yao in the same sequence of the external and internal trigram have responding connection. Good ying is the Yin and Yang respond together.

If we take the second, third and fourth, we got a new trigram which is called mutual Gua. Similarly, we can get another mutual Gua by the third, fourth and fifth.

The relation among the Five Elements are also exist in the external, internal and mutual trigram according to their element properties.

# Table of 64 Gua

| | 天 | 澤 | 火 | 雷 | 風 | 水 | 山 | 地 |
|---|---|---|---|---|---|---|---|---|
| 地 | 否 | 萃 | 晉 | 豫 | 觀 | 比 | 剝 | 坤 |
| 山 | 遯 | 咸 | 旅 | 小過 | 漸 | 蹇 | 艮 | 謙 |
| 水 | 訟 | 困 | 未濟 | 解 | 渙 | 坎 | 蒙 | 師 |
| 風 | 姤 | 大過 | 鼎 | 恆 | 巽 | 井 | 蠱 | 升 |
| 雷 | 無妄 | 隨 | 噬嗑 | 震 | 益 | 屯 | 頤 | 復 |
| 火 | 同人 | 革 | 離 | 豐 | 家人 | 既濟 | 賁 | 明夷 |
| 澤 | 履 | 兌 | 睽 | 歸妹 | 中孚 | 節 | 損 | 臨 |
| 天 | 乾 | 夬 | 大有 | 大壯 | 小畜 | 需 | 大畜 | 泰 |

All Gua are discussed in order from top to bottom, left to right

# Table of Numbers in 64 Gua

六十四卦方圖數字圖

| | Kun | Gen | Kan | Xun | Zhen | Li | Dui | Qian |
|---|---|---|---|---|---|---|---|---|
| 乾 1 | 1 8 | 1 7 | 1 6 | 1 5 | 1 4 | 1 3 | 1 2 | 1 1 |
| 兌 2 | 2 8 | 2 7 | 2 6 | 2 5 | 2 4 | 2 3 | 2 2 | 2 1 |
| 離 3 | 3 8 | 3 7 | 3 6 | 3 5 | 3 4 | 3 3 | 3 2 | 3 1 |
| 震 4 | 4 8 | 4 7 | 4 6 | 4 5 | 4 4 | 4 3 | 4 2 | 4 1 |
| 巽 5 | 5 8 | 5 7 | 5 6 | 5 5 | 5 4 | 5 3 | 5 2 | 5 1 |
| 坎 6 | 6 8 | 6 7 | 6 6 | 6 5 | 6 4 | 6 3 | 6 2 | 6 1 |
| 艮 7 | 7 8 | 7 7 | 7 6 | 7 5 | 7 4 | 7 3 | 7 2 | 7 1 |
| 坤 8 | 8 8 | 8 7 | 8 6 | 8 5 | 8 4 | 8 3 | 8 2 | 8 1 |

# 1/1. Qian is Heaven Creative

乾為天

## Significance:
As Heaven's creative movement is ever vigorous, so must a gentleman ceaselessly strive.

## Suggestion:
Dragon is flying over the sky, good reputation and prosperous. Take the opportunity and achieve the goal.

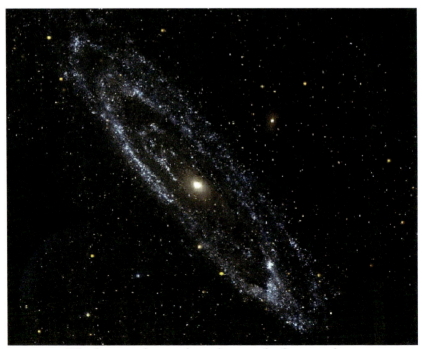

The heaven is moving vigorously for creation.

天澤履

# 1/2. Lyu
# Sky and Lake
# Treading Carefully

## Significance:
The weak meet the strong, tread carefully as it will be difficult and risky to go forward.

## Suggestion:
It will be comfortable after exertion, peaceful after threatening. Be nice and don't hurry. Panic will finish quickly.

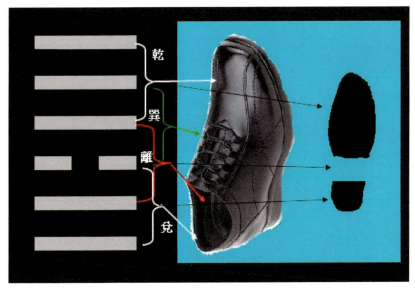

Lyu literally means shoes

天火同人

# 1/3. Tong Ren
# Sky and Fire
# Together with People

### Significance:
Honest and co-operative people get together.

### Suggestion:
Lucky and auspicious. Good opportunity to work with other people in peace. Good chance for promotion.

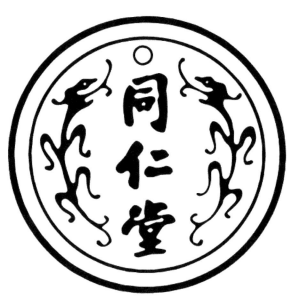

## Sign of Tong Ren Tang

# 1/4. Wu Wang
# Sky and Thunder
# No Untruth

## Significance:
Strength above with thunder below, big rumble, and big warning against untruths.

## Suggestion:
Be honest and sincere. Bad behavior will cause punishment and misfortune.

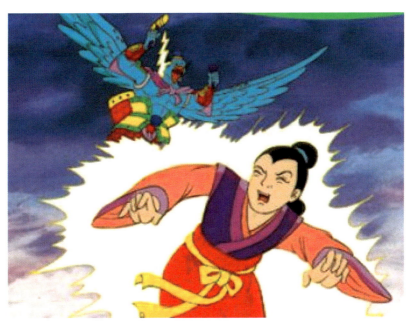

The god of thunder punishes the ignorant liars.

# 1/5. Gou
# Sky and Wind
# Encountering

天 風 姤

## Significance:
Wind intrudes everywhere and discovers what it encounters.

## Suggestion:
Yin is arising even though now it is weak. Yang is fading even though it is strong now. Be careful for what you do, nothing is so easy.

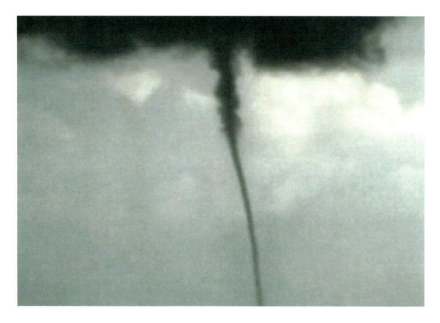

Wind goes everywhere

天 水 訟

# 1/6. Song
# Sky and Water
# Contention

## Significance:
Sky is going up, water is running down. Their destiny's are in contention.

## Suggestion:
What is going on does not agree with you and will make things difficult.  Watch out for traps.

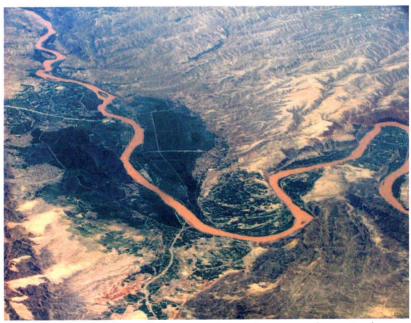

The sky turns towards the west and the river runs down to the east

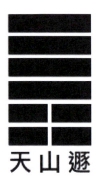

# 1/7. Dun
# Sky and Mountain
# Retreat

天山遯

## Significance:
Sky is escaping. Yin advances, while Yang retreats.

## Suggestion:
It is a good situation for the mean but not good for the kind. Step back and take time for self improvement.

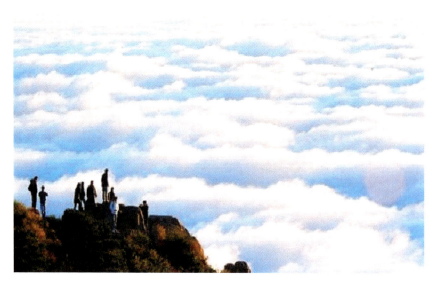

Dun means to escape

# 1/8. Pi
# Sky and Earth
# Stagnation

### Significance:

No interaction between the heaven Qi and earth Qi causing stagnation.

### Suggestion:

Disharmonized relationship between superior and inferior. Things are stagnated, wait for the harmony.

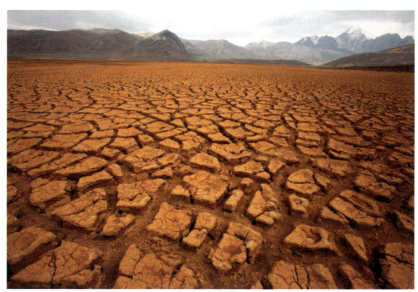

Pi means stagnation due to lack of intercourse
between the sky and the Earth and there is no rain.

澤天夬

# 2/1. Guai
# Marsh and Sky
# Outburst

## Significance:
Water hangs over the sky like a rain cloud that will can burst at any moment. The only Yin will disappear.

## Suggestion:
Even now it is not bad, the difficulties are forming. Try to avoid ego and arguments.

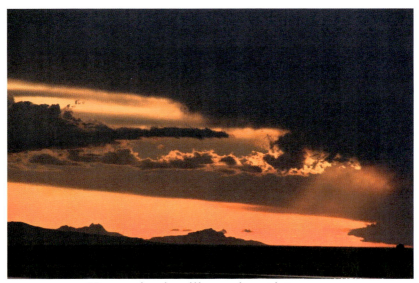

Heavy clouds will soon burst into pour

# 2/2. Dui is Marsh
# Joy

兑 為 澤

## Significance:

Joyful scenery of lake and marsh mirrors the moon.

## Suggestion:

Life is full of happiness and sadness, applause and criticism. Keep doing what is right and end with satisfaction.

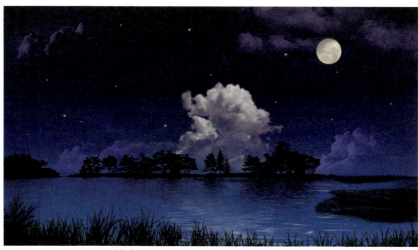

Beautiful scenery makes people feel happy

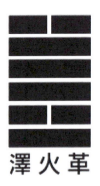

澤火革

# 2/3. Ge
# Marsh and Fire
# Revolution

## Significance:
Dui is also metal which is being forged into weapons for revolution.

## Suggestion:
Discard the old and adapt to the new in the process of change.

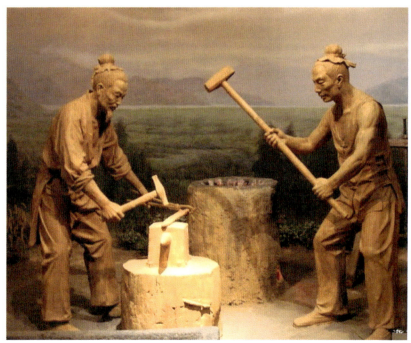

To build weapons for the revolution

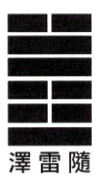

# 2/4. Sui
# Marsh and Thunder
# Following

澤 雷 隨

## Significance:

Lei is wood which floats on the river and follows the running water.

## Suggestion:

Good sign for the new things. It is a profitable opportunity to work with others. Try to avoid hesitation and acting solely on one's own opinion.

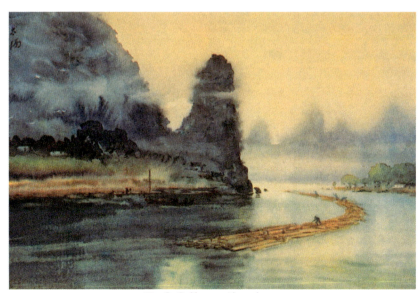

Raft follows the river

# 2/5. Da Guo
# Marsh and Wind
# Big in Excess

## Significance:
Heavy middle is too much for the weak ends. Lei is also trees which are merged by flood. Such an excess may collapse any time soon.

## Suggestion:
Heavy burden and stress are too much for one to carry.

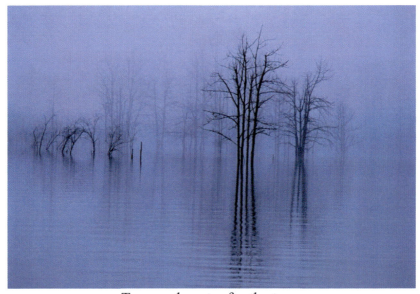

Too much water for the trees

澤水困

# 2/6. Kun
# Marsh and Water
# Trapped

### Significance:
Water disappeared and is trapped under the river, nothing survived.

### Suggestion:
Poverty and unfavorable situation.

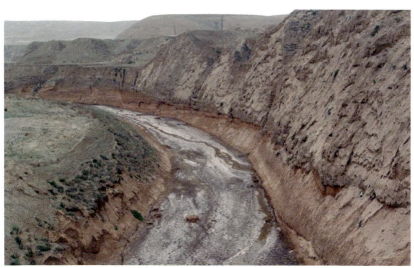

Everything is trapped in the dried river bed

# 2/7. Xian
# Marsh and Mountain
# Mutual Attraction

澤山咸

## Significance:

Mutual attraction between a girl (Ze) and a boy (Gen) will lead to marriage.

## Suggestion:

It is a lucky time. Do not indulge into relationship and ignore other more important things.

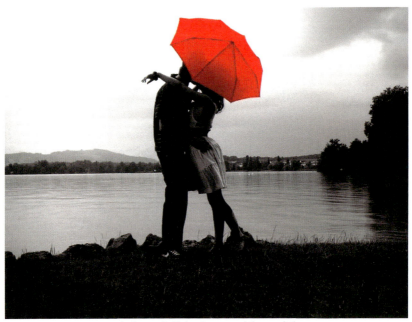

A boy fell in love with a girl

# 2/8. Cui
# Marsh and Earth
# Gathering

澤 地 萃

## Significance:
Marsh on the rich land nourishes all the plants which gather together.

## Suggestion:
Prosperous and bright future with support of the superiors. Try to avoid financial argument.

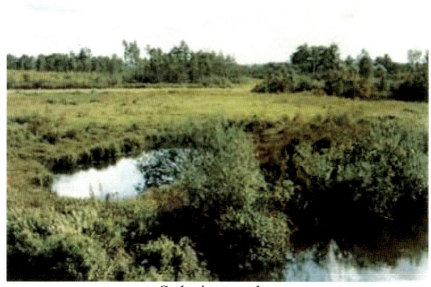

Gathering together

# 3/1. Da You
# Fire and Sky
# Great Possession

火天大有

## Significance:
The Sun shines the earth. The five Yang compete for one Yin.

## Suggestion:
All the best for luck and prosperity, but even the best situation won't last forever.

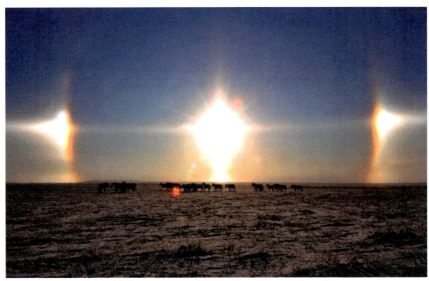

As if there were three Suns over the sky

# 3/2. Kui
# Fire and March
# Estrangement

火澤睽

## Significance:

Li is a young lady with fire nature flares up; Zui is a girl with water nature runs down.  It is trouble for them when living together.

## Suggestion:

Everything is difficult and no luck. Fire and water do not agree to each other.

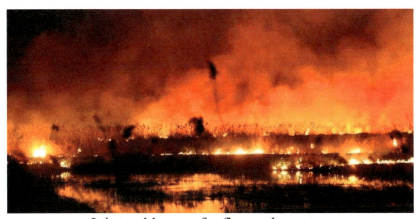

It is troublesome for fire on the water.

火澤睽

# 3/3. Li is Fire
# Sunlight

## Significance:
Sunlight is bright but without a shape and not solid.

## Suggestion:
Do not push forward by the attractive grand view like sunlight.

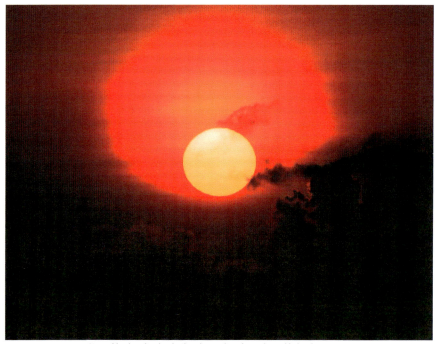

Sunlight is bright but lack of solid shape.

106

# 3/4. Shi Ke
# Fire and Thunder
# Biting Through

火雷噬嗑

## Significance:

The stuff between the two rows of teeth must be bit through for the mouth to close.

## Suggestion:

There are so many obstacles and arguments have to be removed by following regulation and policies. Do not be misled by small profit.

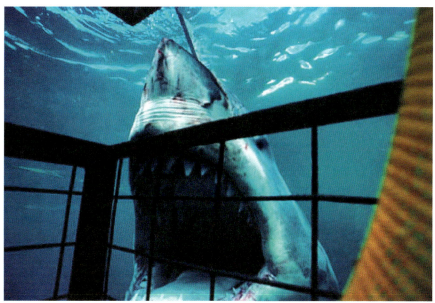

A strong bite

# 3/5. Ding
# Fire and Wind
# Cauldron

## Significance:

Xun is wood with fire burning above for cooking in a Cauldron.

## Suggestion:

Cauldron was used for ceremonies of a new event. It is high time to start a new project. Be careful not to have a lawsuit.

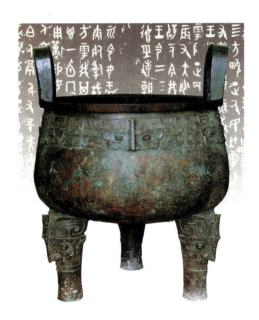

A huge cooking pot

# 3/6. Wei Ji
# Fire and Water
# Accomplishment Not Yet
# Realized

## Significance:
Fire flares up and water runs down naturally. There is no intercourse between the two and no accomplishment can be realized.

## Suggestion:
It is not a lucky time. Be patient and do not give up. Success will come eventually.

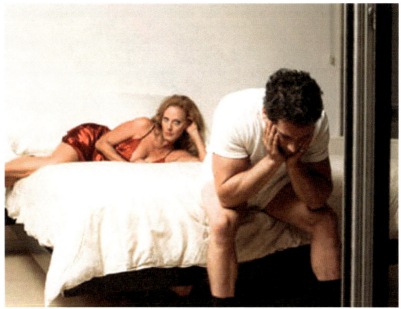

There is no intercourse between Yin and Yang.

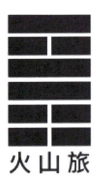

# 3/7. Liu
# Fire and Mountain
# Traveling

### Significance:
Fire burning up the mountain, travelling forward like a wanderer with no fixed place to stay.

### Suggestion:
In an unsure situation, keep the faith, listen to others or there might be bad things to come.

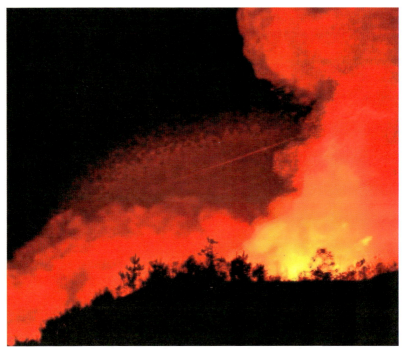

Fire has no place to stay after burning.

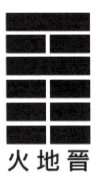

# 3/8. Jin
# Fire and Earth
# Progress

火地晉

### Significance:
The sun rising above the horizon, progressively lighting the earth.

### Suggestion:
It is lucky signs for career, reputation and fortune.

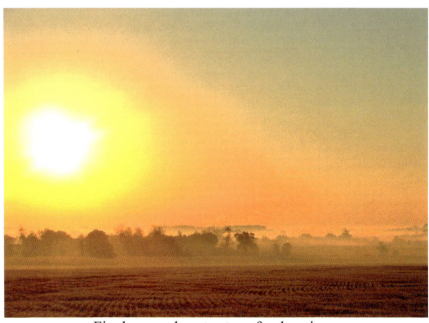

Fire has no place to stay after burning.

# 4/1. Da Zhuang
# Thunder and Sky
# Great Strength

## Significance:

Great strength in thunder with its loud sound, brightness and vibration.

## Suggestion:

It is strong but it is close to the end. Soon it will be quiet. Be peaceful or it is easy to end up with failure. Too cold so warm.

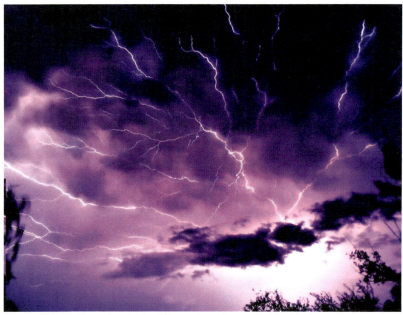

Thunder is brilliant but does not last long.

# 4/2. Gui Mei
# Thunder and Marsh
# Relationship

## Significance:

Zhen is the elder brother, Dui is the younger sister, and the young having to follow the old is an unfavorable relationship.

## Suggestion:

It is an abnormal relationship from which, benefit first, risk and trouble will follow.

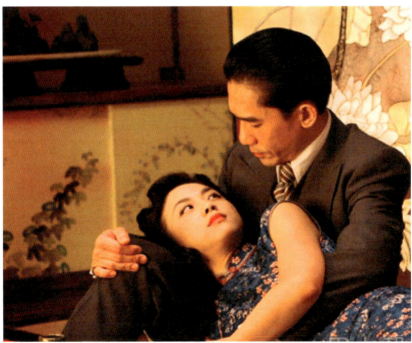

Elder man and young girl do not match.

# 4/3. Feng
# Thunder and Fire
# Prosperity

雷火豐

## Significance:

The view of thunder and lightening under the sun is grand and prosperous.

## Suggestion:

It is good enough. Do not be greedy. Happiness is from self-satisfaction.

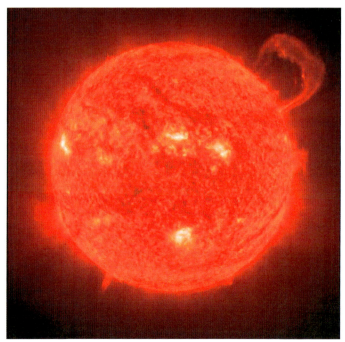

Grand view of thunder on the Sun

震為雷

# 4/4. Lei is Thunder
# Shock

## Significance:
Heavy thunders vibrates the earth to make changes. Only a shock and no danger.

## Suggestion:
There are uncertain changes hidden in the grand view.

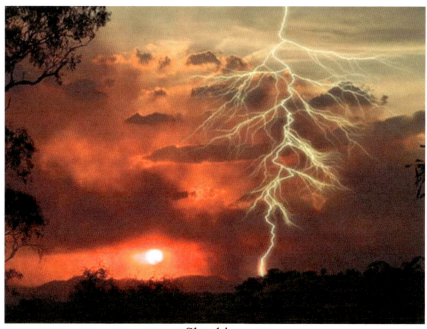

Shocking

# 4/5. Heng
# Thunder and Wind
# Constancy

雷風恆

## Significance:

Zhen's tendency is outward; Xun's tendency is inward. This is the constant way for a couple.

## Suggestion:

To keep the constancy is good choice. To make unexpected changes is risky.

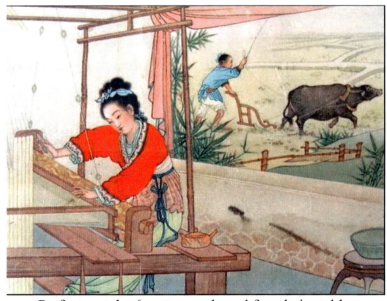

Perfect match of mature male and female is stable.

# 4/6. Jie
# Thunder and Water
# Release

雷 水 解

### Significance:
In spring, thunder releases the ice and awakens all the creatures.

### Suggestion:
Take action quickly when the opportunity comes. Leave the difficult place and find a new place to start.

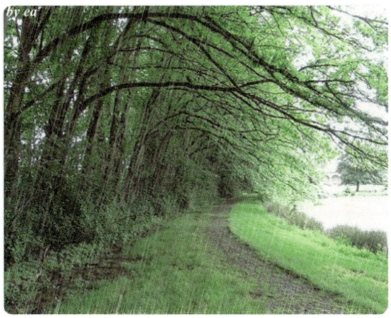

Dryness is released by the thunder and rain.

# 4/7. Xiao Guo:
# Thunder and Mountain
# Small Excess

## Significance:

Thunder behind the far mountains. It is a small excess when the sound and light arrives.

## Suggestion:

Nothing is smooth. Do minor business instead of big investment. Avoid causing argument for small mistake (excess).

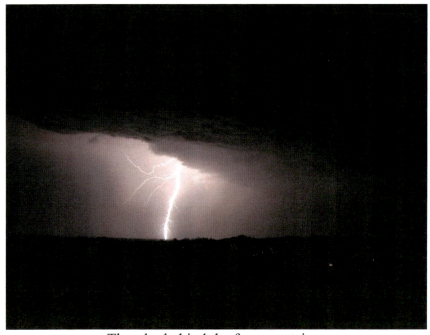

Thunder behind the far mountains.

# 4/8. Yu
# Thunder and Earth
# Enthusiasm

雷 地 豫

## Significance:

Thunder awakens the earth, Yang is activated, all plants are happy and enthusiastic.

## Suggestion:

Supported by superiors, everything is lucky and peaceful. Prepare well to start.

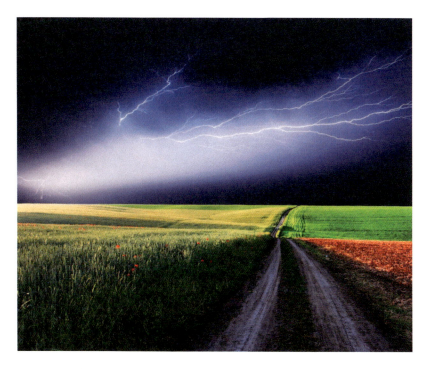

All the plants are happy when there is thunder.

# 5/1. Xiao Xu:
# Wind and Sky
# Small Accumulation

## Significance:

Wind in the sky, the small accumulation is limited. It is not the time, wait for larger accumulation.

## Suggestion:

The situation is not steady and arguments cannot be solved in the short term. Be patient and wait for better chance.

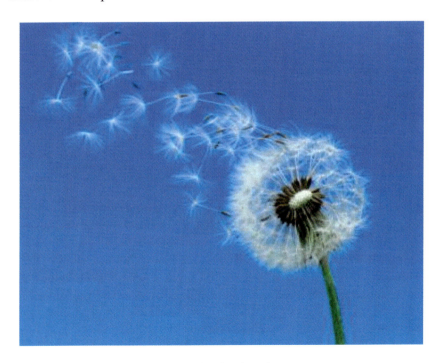

Not a lot in the air

# 5/2. Zhong Fu
# Wind and Marsh
# Inner Truth

風澤中孚

### Significance:
Water in the lake responds to wind with inner truth.

### Suggestion:
Be truthful, sincere and trustworthy. Bad intention leads to danger.

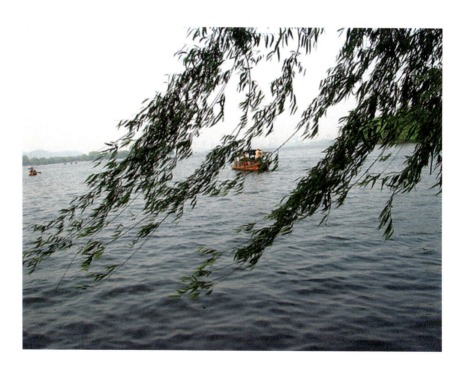

Waving with wind

# 5/3. Jia Ren
# Wind and Fire
# Family

風火家人

## Significance:

Family is a place with fire in the furnace and wind make the fire strong. All the family members work together with whole heart and soul.

## Suggestion:

It is a sign of peace and luck. It will be successful to co-operate with others.

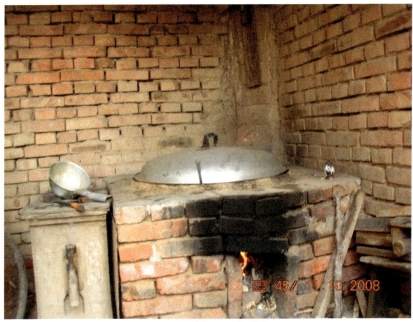

Stove with a wind box

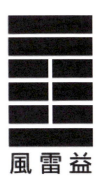

# 5/4. Yi
# Wind and Thunder
# Increase

風雷益

## Significance:
Strong wind with thunder, the synergy of the elder brother and the elder sister, both reputation and benefits are increased.

## Suggestion:
It is at good time. Success will be achieved by support from noble people. It is more meaningful to help others.

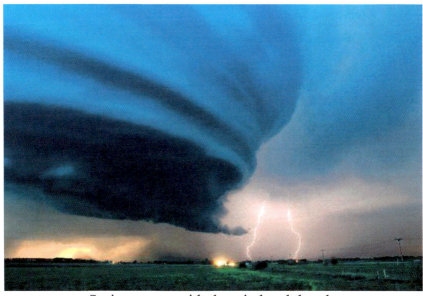

Spring comes with the wind and thunder

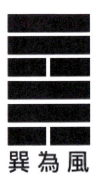

巽 為 風

# 5/5. Xun is Wind
# Gentle Penetration

## Significance:

Wind gently penetrates everywhere it goes. If the regulations and laws work in this way, it is good for the society.

## Suggestion:

Try to be flexible in dealing with difficulties, by peacefully according to the situation.

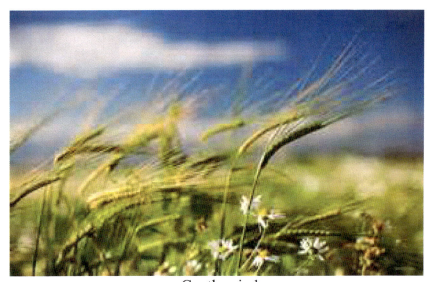

Gentle wind

# 5/6. Huan
# Wind and Water
# Dispersion

風水渙

## Significance:

Wind disperses the ice and water. Water is running around.

## Suggestion:

Difficulties will be dispersed with good result, though there are risks. Avoid being stubborn.

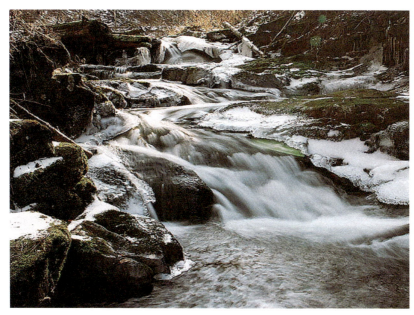

Ice is dissolving and water runs in dispersion

# 5/7. Jian
# Wind and Mountain
# Gradual Development

風山漸

## Significance:

Everything has to develop gradually like trees growing on mountains.

## Suggestion:

Make a good foundation, slow and steady leads to a bright future. Prevent mistakes in relationship and writing.

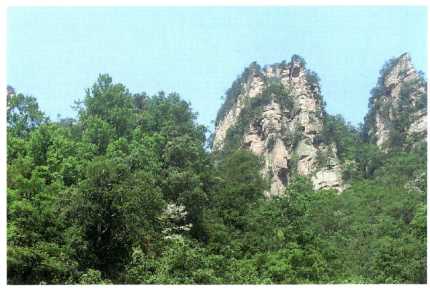

Trees grow on the mountains

126

風 地 觀

# 5/8. Guan
# Wind and Earth
# Watching

## Significance:
Wind travels over the earth as if watching over the land. Yin is increasing and Yang is decreasing. Watch for negative changes.

## Suggestion:
Watch carefully in stressful and changing situations. Avoid negative temptations.

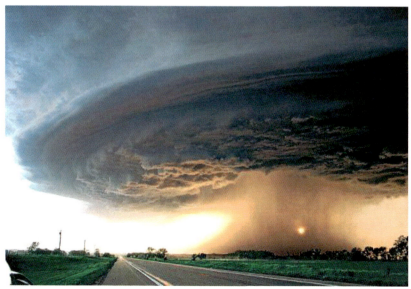

Whirling Wind

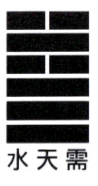

水天需

# 6/1. Xu
# Water and Sky
# Making the Most of
# Waiting

## Significance:
Clouds hang over the sky and the rain will pour down any time.
Make the most of waiting for the rain.

## Suggestion:
It is wise to wait for the best time to start. It is risky to start without
careful preparation.

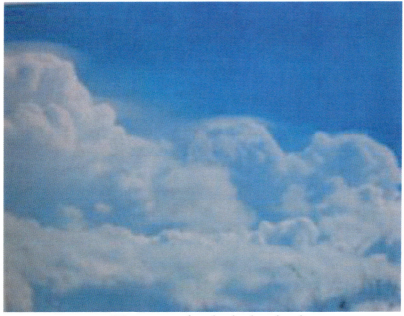

Water over the sky is the clouds.

# 6/2. Jie
# Water and Marsh
# Frugality

水澤節

## Significance:

Water in the pond should be used with frugality. If the water goes above the pond it is also a waste.

## Suggestion:

Self-control is necessary for those who have great ambition.

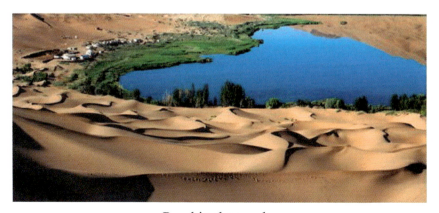

Pond in the sands

# 6/3. Ji Ji
# Water and Fire
# Successful
# Accomplishment

## Significance:
Water goes down to be steamed by the fire; fire goes up to heat the water. This is successful accomplishment.

## Suggestion:
It is a sign of success of both reputation and business. Be aware that unfavorable things follow success.

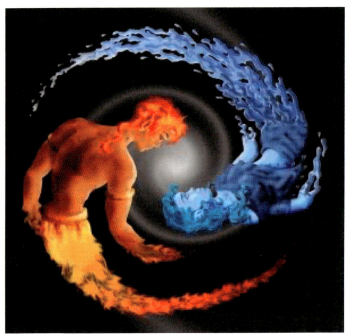

Good communication between Yin and Yang

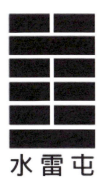

水雷屯

# 6/4. Zun
# Water and Thunder
# Initial Difficulty

Significance:
Initially, the first step is full of difficulty.

Suggestion:
Moving forward firmly in dilemma. After the initial difficulty, things will go well.

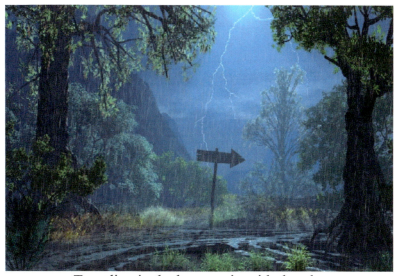

Traveling in the heavy rain with thunder

# 6/5. Jing
# Water and Wind
# A Well

水風井

## Significance:

A plant takes water from the earth like a well replenishes those who draw from it.

## Suggestion:

A well passively waits for others to take water from it, rather than actively supply water to their doors.

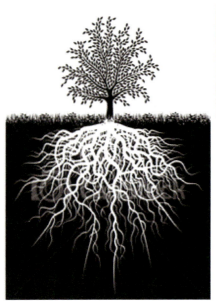

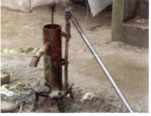

A old style pump well

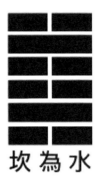

# 6/6. Kan is Water Abyss

坎 為 水

## Significance:

Surrounded by an abyss of water, nowhere is safe whether going forward or back.

## Suggestion:

Risk is everywhere. Avoid arguments and be optimistic.

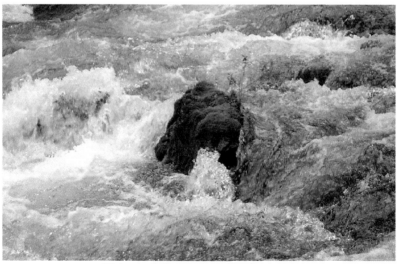

This rock is not a safe place to stay.

# 6/7. Jian
# Mountains and Water
# Obstructions to Progress

水山蹇

## Significance:

It is difficult to decide where to proceed with deep water obstructing in front and high mountains behind.

## Suggestion:

When there are obstructions to progress, be careful when taking the chance of facing the risk.

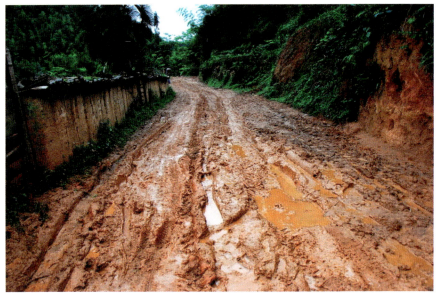

A difficult mountain road

水 地 比

# 6/8. Bi
# Water and Earth
# Harmony

### Significance:
One Yang governs five Yin in good position. This is harmony.

### Suggestion:
Do not hesitate in taking quick action with support of superior in this favorable situation.

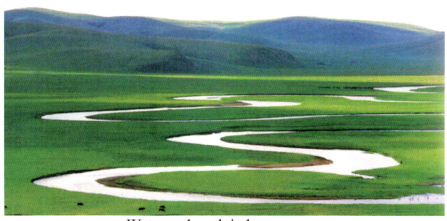

Water and earth in harmony

# 7/1. Da Xu
# Mountains and Sky
# Great Accumulating

## Significance:
The mountain is so big it seems as if a great accumulation above the sky.

## Suggestion:
Achievement is grounded in a strong foundation but is not possible from arrogance.

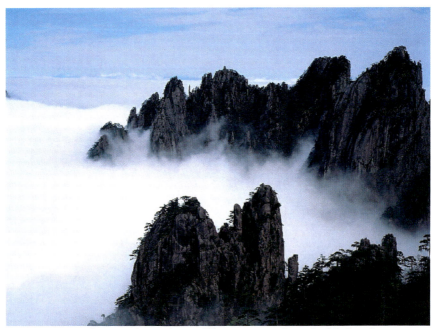

Mountains are huge but still not enough to hold the sky.

# 7/2. Sun
# Mountain and Marsh
# Decrease

山澤損

### Significance:
Mountain is high, river is deep. Increase is from what decreases.

### Suggestion:
It is not favorable in decrease. Benefit will come from the lost.

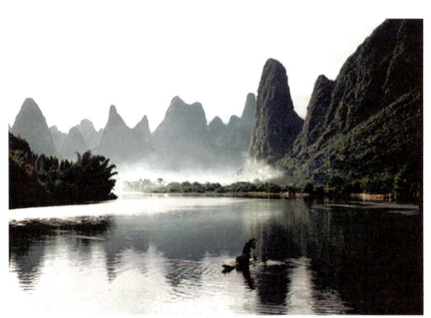

Deep water nourishes high mountains.

# 7/3. Bi
# Mountain and Fire
# Decoration

山火賁

## Significance:

The sun went down behind the mountains. It looks as beautiful as a decoration. Darkness will conquer the sunset soon.

## Suggestion:

Beauty is skin deep like temporary sunset. Improve internal beauty by self-improvement.

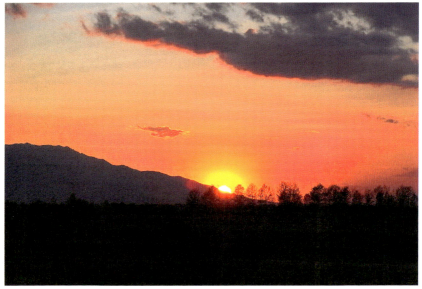

Beautiful sunset

# 7/4. Yi
# Mountain and Thunder
# Nourishment

山雷頤

## Significance:
Symbol of a mouth relates with diet, nourishment and speech.

## Suggestion:
Be mindful of the food you eat and the words you use.

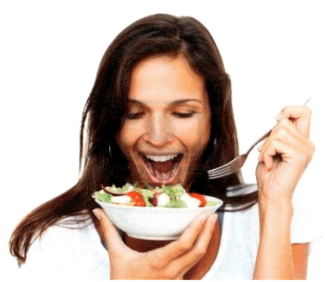

You are what you eat.

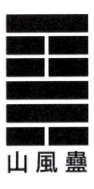

# 7/5. Gu
# Mountain and Wind
# Poison

山風蠱

## Significance:
Air in the mountains lacks circulation and becomes poisonous.

## Suggestion:
Toxic situation that needs to be remedied or it will develop into chaos.

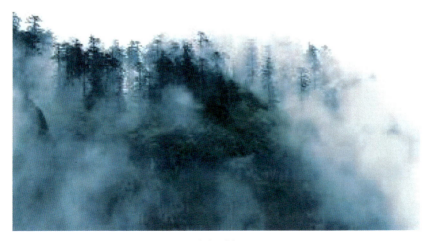

A world of insects

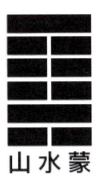

# 7/6. Meng
# Mountian and Water
# Ignorance

山水蒙

## Significance:

Ignorance before the mist clears from in front of the mountain.

## Suggestion:

Ignorance is not a problem if one is willing to listen and learn from the wise.

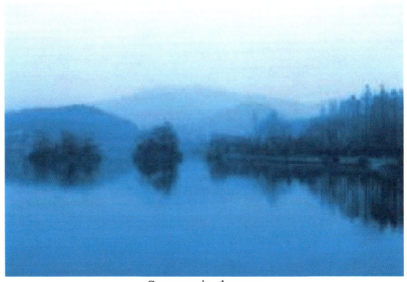

Scenery in dreams

# 7/7. Gen is Mountain Stilling

艮為山

## Significance:
Mountains block the way thereby keeping things still.

## Suggestion:
The road is blocked. Do not make progress until one finds the way.

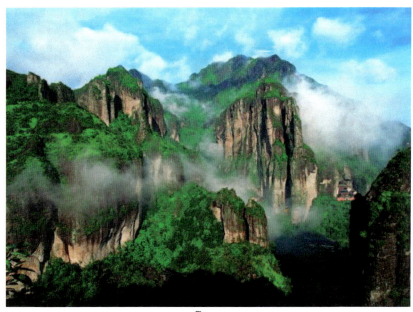

Stop

山地剝

# 7/8. Bo
# Mountain and Earth
# Decomposing

### Significance:
Stones falling off the decomposing mountain. Five Yin drive the only Yang away. No justice.

### Suggestion:
Bad luck. Be careful of bad people.

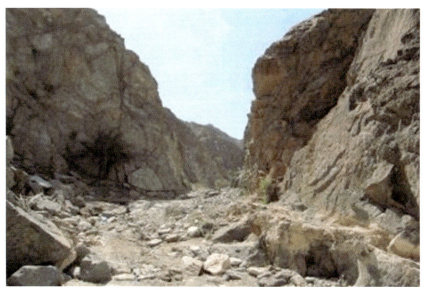

A peeled mountain

143

# 8/1. Tai
# Earth and Sky
# Overall Harmony

地天泰

## Significance:

It is a sign of overall harmony of the Qi of Yin and Yang have perfect interaction without stagnation.

## Suggestion:

All are in favor. Rely on self and not on others. Beware of sadness hidden in happiness.

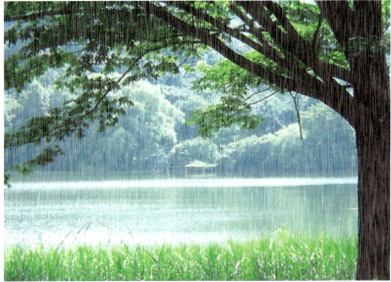

Raining is the sign for interaction between heaven and the Earth.

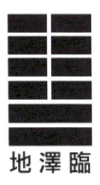

# 8/2. Lin
# Earth and Marsh
# Approaching

地澤臨

## Significance:
Earth and marsh approach each other to oversee keeping a good environment for all creatures.

## Suggestion:
All are going smoothly and harmoniously towards the bright future. No rush needed.

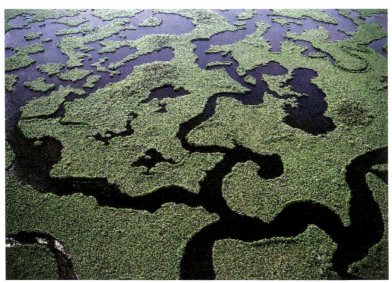

Marsh is the lung of the Earth.

# 8/3. Ming Yi
# Earth and Fire
# Brightness Hidden

## Significance:

The sun is going down the horizon. The earth looses brightness and becomes dark.

## Suggestion:

All is not going smoothly with the problems darkness brings. In this confusing situation, wait quietly for the opportunity.

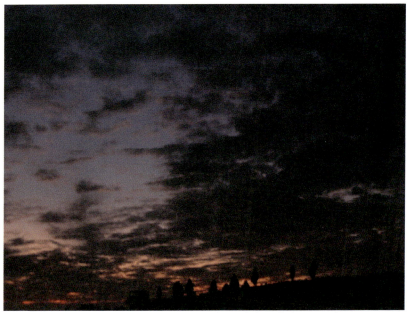

The Sun moved to the other side of the Earth.

地雷復

# 8/4. Fu
# Earth and Thunder
# Returning

## Significance:
Thunder awakens the earth. One Yang returns, spring is returning.

## Suggestion:
Good beginning, follow what is going on and no hurry.

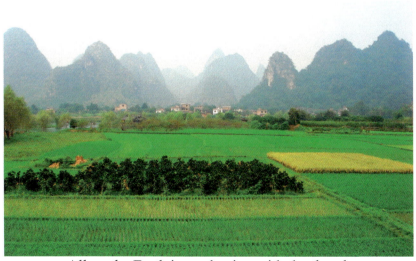

All on the Earth is awakening with the thunder.

# 8/5. Sheng
# Earth and Wind
# Ascending

地風升

## Significance:
Plants are ascending from the earth and growing bigger.


## Suggestion:
Good sign for both reputation and business.

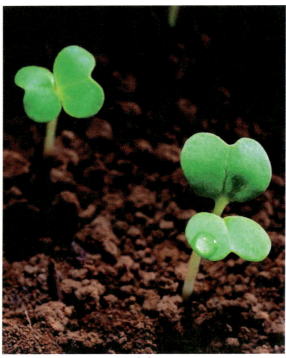

Arising

地水師

# 8/6. Shi
# Earth and Water
# Army

## Significance:

The real army is in the population like the water under the earth.
War is not good for either side.

## Suggestion:

Difficult situation in which one should firmly prepare for the potential
enemy.

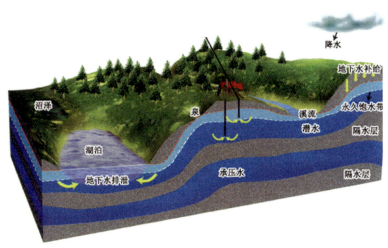

A hidden river

# 8/7. Qian
# Earth Mountain
# Modesty

地山謙

## Significance:
Great modesty should be like the heaven hidden under the earth.


## Suggestion:
Peace and safety come from modesty. Future is bright.

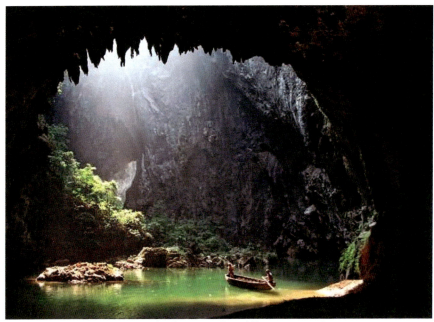

A mountain in cave is still a mountain.

坤為地

# 8/8. Kun is Earth Receptive

## Significance:

Earth receptivity holds all creatures and with great virtue and kindness.

## Suggestion:

Quietly yielding is more powerful than fast progress.

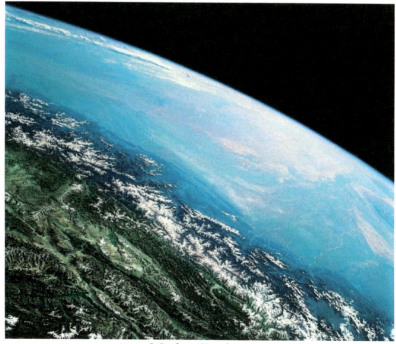

Mother Earth

# 8 QIAN KUN, MODEL OF THE TIME AND SPACE

Qian Kun is a Chinese word which means the universe. We can see this word was from the two trigrams, Qian and Kun. To study the Yi Jing, we always start with those two Gua because they are the doors of Yi Jing. Depending on the location of Qian and Kun in the circular sequence of 64 hexagrams, there are three different Yi: Zhou Yi（周易）, Mountain Yi（连山易）and Earth Yi（归藏易）. Today the most popular Yi is Zhou Yi. The other two Yi have become secrets.

Confucius started to study Yi in his fifties and was attracted by its beauty. He wrote a book "Ten Wings" and made Yi a philosophy system. Yi was developed through three sages Fuxi, King Wen and Confucius and in three different times became the complete system known as Yi Jing.

Yi, 易，the top part is the character of the Sun and the bottom is the character of the Moon. The Sun and the Moon represent the change of day and night; this change is constant, this change is steady and this change is simple, because it is the great Dao of Yin and Yang.

So the Yi system is a model of time and space in the universe. With 64 codes and their sequences, Yi summarizes the rules and principles that work throughout the entire universe.

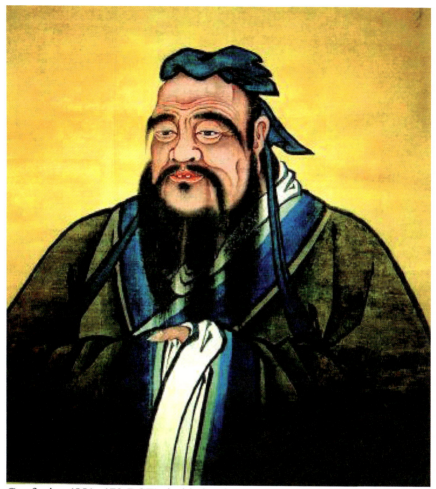

Confucius (551–479 BCE), in his book "Ten Wings", wrote texts for all the hexagrams and each yao. These are explanations to the sequences of the 64 Gua. From his work, Yi subsequently became a complete philosophy system.

Qian is a pure Yang Gua with 6 Yang yao symbolized 6 Long, Chinese dragons, to govern the world:

Bottom:  hiding Long, do not act
Second:  appearing Long, ready to act, but limited
Third:  alert Long, must do everything cautiously and prudently
Fourth:  leaping Long, act with the timing and reach to the sky
Fifth:  flying Long, carry out his aspirations and benefit all
Top:  over-acting Long, regret for reaching the end

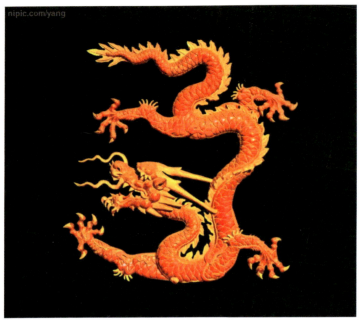

Chinese dragon is a spiritual animal with characters of 9 real animals' parts. Chinese dragon can be big and small, can fly and swim. It is the symbol of royal family. Chinese dragon is totally different from the western dragon. It is better to keep the original name "Long" to avoid misunderstanding.

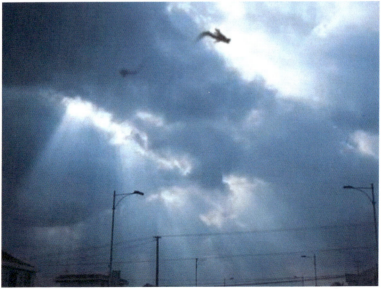

Long is a mysterious animal. It is believed to be real.

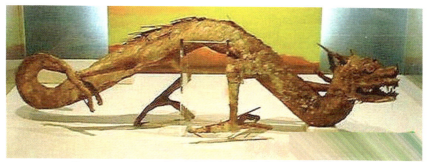

Long specimen kept in a Temple in Osaka, Japan

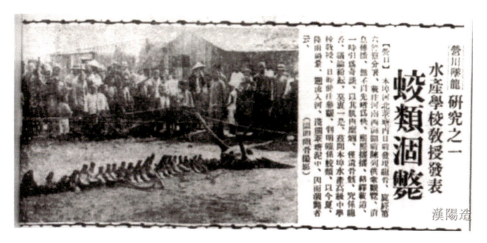

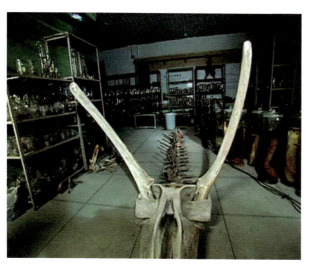

In 1934, a living long was found in Ying Kou. It disappeared in a heavy rain and 20 days later, the same long was found dead on another spot 10 kilometers away. The skeleton is now kept in Dalian.

Kun is pure Yin Gua with 6 Yin yao which is designated to sustain and submit to Qian:

Bottom: step onto the frosted ground and hard ice, be careful

Second: straight, square and big, to follow whatever that is

Third:  hide the brilliance

Fourth: hiding in a tied up bag

Fifth:  the yellow costume, auspicious

Top:   fighting Long, blood blends together

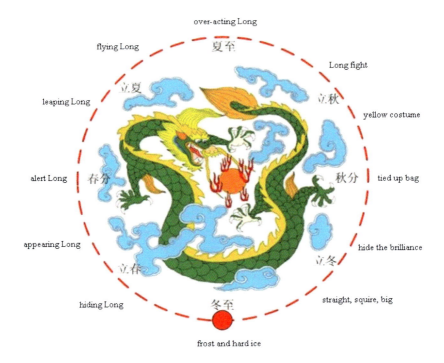

Qian is Yang, Kun is Yin, and they are in one Taiji circle.

The instinct of Qian is creative and perseverant; the instinct of Kun is submissive and receptive.

Qian is Long which is flying in the sky; Kun is female horse which is galloping on the ground.

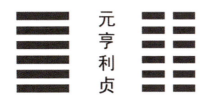

The four virtues of the heaven are paraphrased by Confucius as 元 (yuan), 亨 (heng), 利(li), 贞(zhen) which are origination, circulation, harmony and correctness. Those four words are magic, when they apply to a Gua, the Gua is the lucky one. Confucius generously gave all the four words to both Qian and Kun.

The four virtues repeat in cycles again and again without an end. The entire universe is progressing forward in spiral forms.

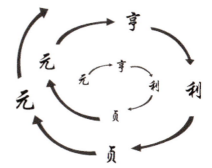

"The mighty origin of Qian! The whole of creation counts on it to initiate; thus it rules the heavens"

"The utmost origin of Kun! The whole creation counts on it to grow, it submissively sustains the will of heaven"

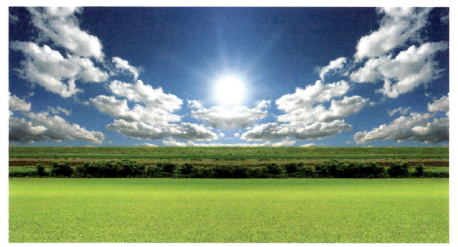

大哉乾元，万物资始，乃统天。至哉坤元，万物资生，乃顺承天

# Pre-natal round diagram of 64 Gua

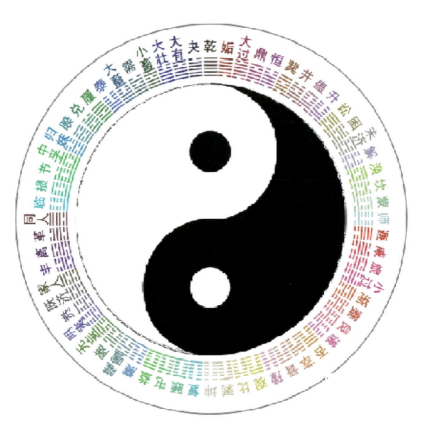

In ancient China, the heaven is round, the Earth is square, so this represents the heaven;

The eight pure Gua (same for the external and internal) are located in the same position as the pre-natal Bagua;

The internal Gua follow the pre-natal numbers and make changes every 8 Gua, the external Gua follow the pre-natal numbers and make changes at each Gua. This is a more detailed pre-natal Bagua.

# Pre-natal square diagram of 64 Gua

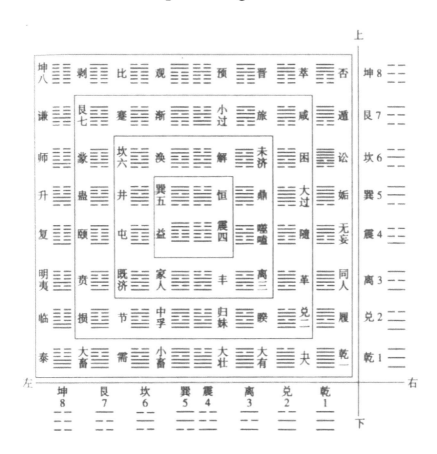

This diagram is square, so represents the Earth. Watch the lower right and upper left corners of the squares. The inner square is where the wind swipes the land with thunder. The second square is the Sun and the Moon spinning over the sky. The third square is the air circulating between mountain and lake. The fourth square is where the Heaven and the Earth are located.

# The pre-natal square and round diagram of 64 Gua

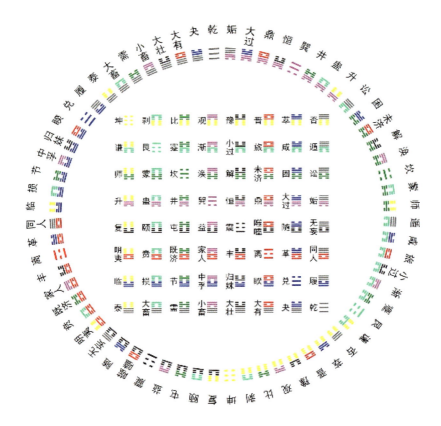

This is the time and space model of the Heaven and the Earth;
The round diagram is the time model. The square is the space model;
The south is Yang for the heaven. The north is Yang for the Earth.

## Post-natal square diagram of 64 Gua

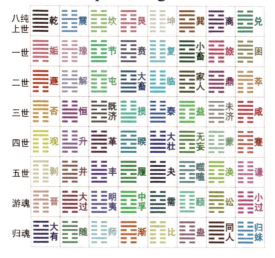

## Post-natal round diagram of 64 Gua

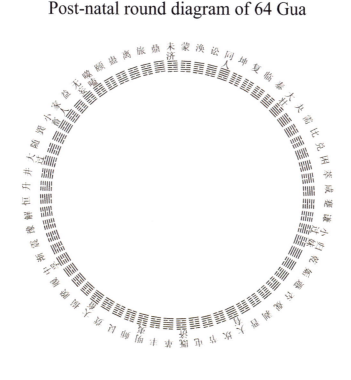

# The Unified Taiji Diagram

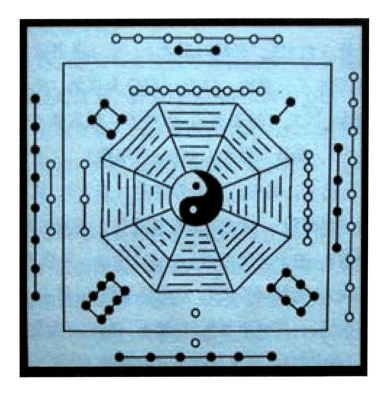

Yi Jing reveals the basic principles of the universe by concepts of space and time, movement and tranquility, Yin and Yang. He Tu, Luo Shu, pre-natal and post-natal Bagua, 64 square and round diagrams are all parts of the information of Taiji. The universe is in absolute movement, also in dynamic balance. The balance is based on the change of Yin and Yang, the change of Yin and Yang is for the balance.

# Meridians and Organs in Unified Taiji System

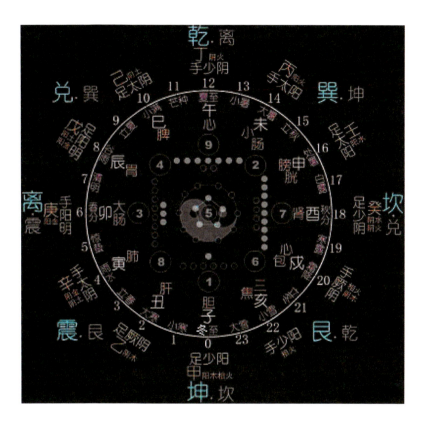

Application of those universal principles to medicine is Chinese medicine, 中医，pronounced as Zhong Yi. Zhong, literally means middle and balance, Yi, means medicine and interesting enough, the same sound as 易 in Yi Jing, and pronunciation of "one" in Chinese which means Taiji. Yi and medicine (Yi) are one (Yi). Is that a coincidence?

In this sense, Chinese medicine is the balance, changing and Taiji medicine.

# 9 ONE CIRCULATING QI

Everything between the Heaven and Earth can be seen as one Qi circulating in cycles. This is the known Taiji which is moving to create Yang and freezing to become Yin. Ascending Qi is Yang; descending Qi is Yin. Yang is the prime power for the circulation; Yin is the pathway of Yang.

"天地之大德曰生"
"The great virtue of Heaven and Earth is creation".

Human is the son of Qi from both Heaven and Earth, so human is also one Qi circulating inside the body which is part of the Qi between the Earth and Heaven. It is the reason why human responds to the Heaven. When this one Qi is circulating within different locations, it shows different properties known as Five Elements. Qi moves everywhere, if we see it at different levels or angles, there are Yin Yang in Yin and Yin Yang in Yang; Yin Yang in Five Elements; Five Elements in Yin and Yang; and Five Elements within each Element.

大道至简，  Great Dao is the simplest.

The simplest medicine is the one Qi medicine.

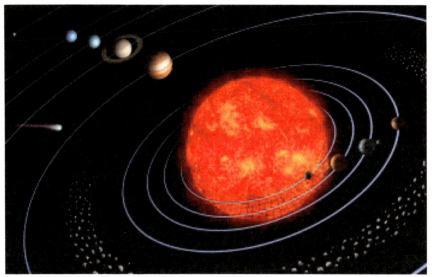

The greatest in the sky is the Sun.

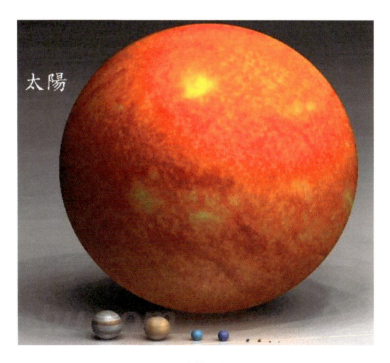

The mass of the Sun occupies 99.8% of the solar system

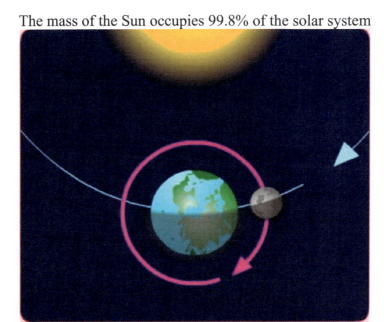

Yin and Yang concept came directly from observing the Sun's movement.

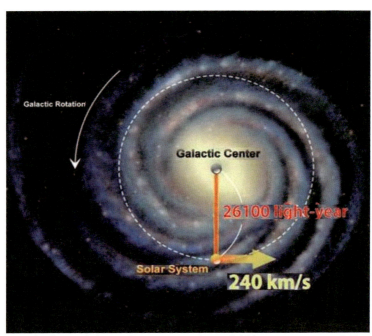

The revolution of the solar system is at 240km per second. It takes

26100 light-years to finish one circle around the galaxy.

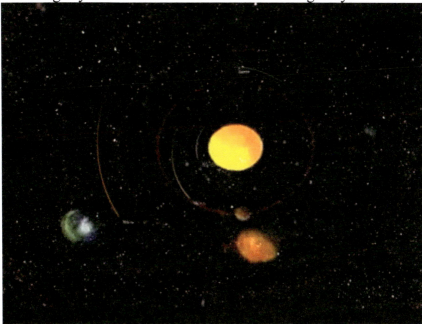

Currently the Sun is spinning forward towards us. It moves toward us with an anticlockwise movement.

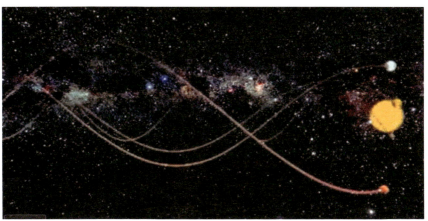

The movement of the solar system is in spiral form.

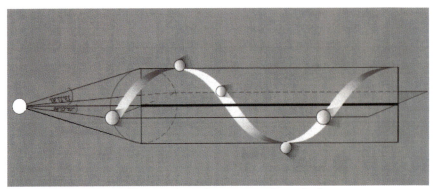

Dynamic solar system in spiral

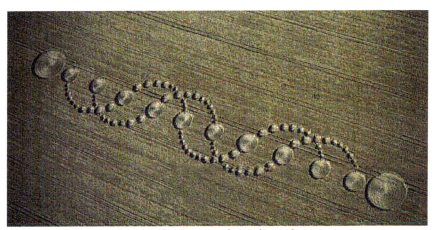

It is a basic pattern for other planets.

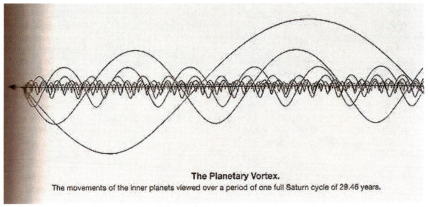

The planetary vortex

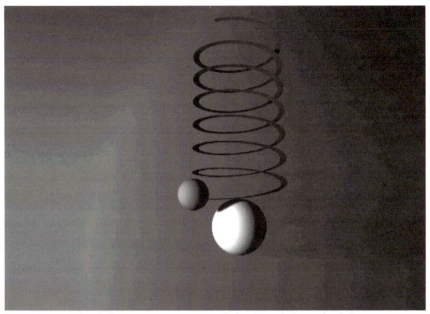

The Moon moves around the Earth in spiral form.

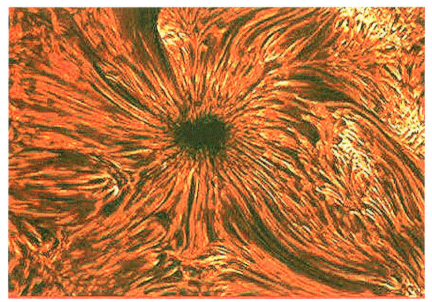

Electricity whirlpool around a sunspot

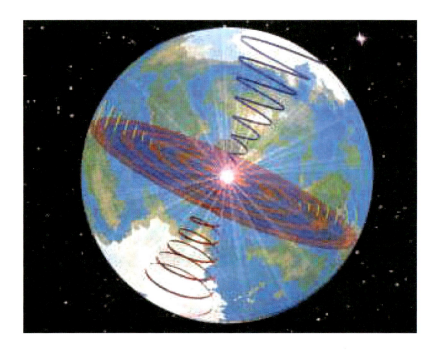

The planetary whirl of the Earth

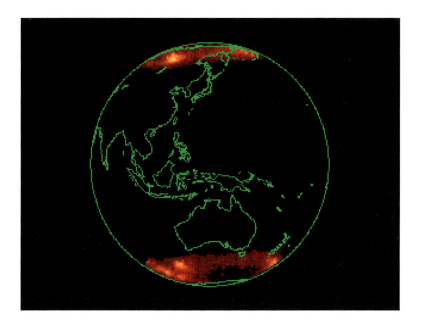

Whirls on two poles of the Earth

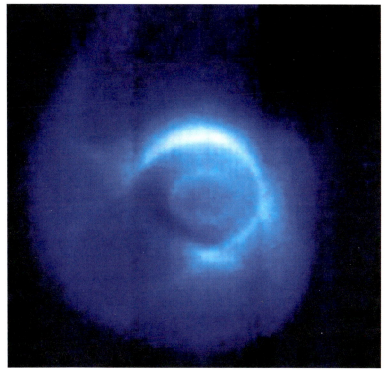

Plasma whirl on north pole

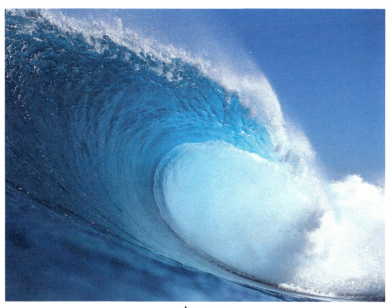

A wave

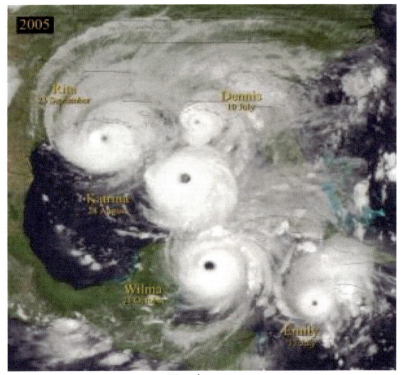

Hurricanes

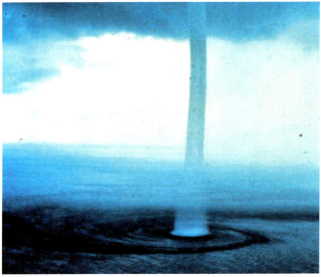

Spiral Tornado

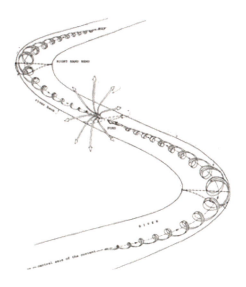

Water current in river

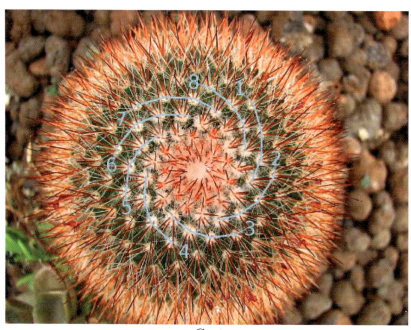

Cactus

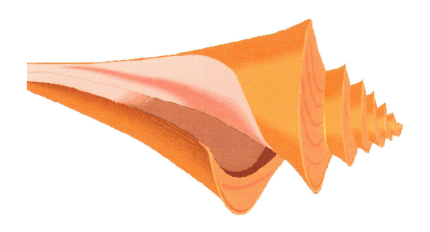

Frozen Spiral Movement

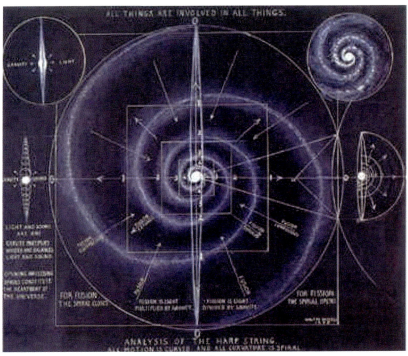

A Vibrating String

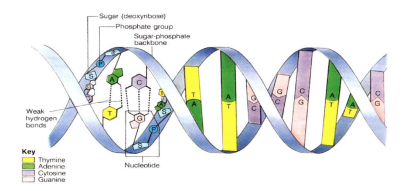

Spiral Structure of DNA

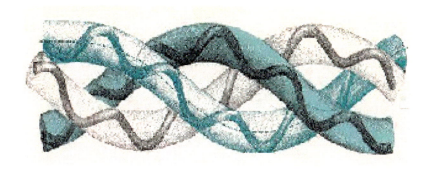

Gelatin

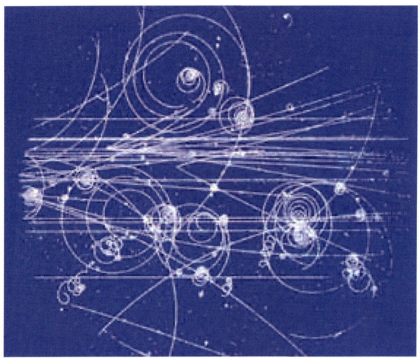

Particle Collision

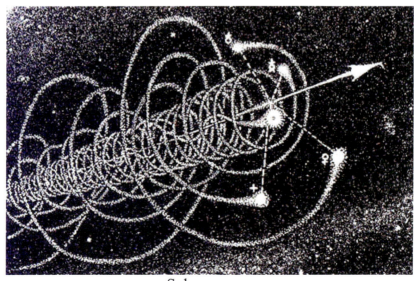

Solar energy

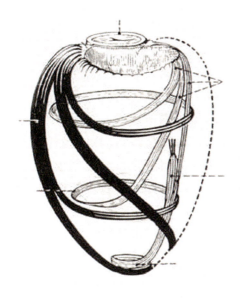

Now we can see, the spiral structure is the basic form of movement in the universe, from the biggest to the smallest, with or without a shape. If the solar energy moves forward like the picture above, let's make a guess. How about the blood moving in the vessels? How about Qi moving in the meridians?

The answer is, Qi should be spinning forward like the solar energy in spiral form. If we see it in front of the arrow, the moving direction should be anticlockwise. If we see it behind, the moving direction should be clockwise. This direction creates centrifugal force which neutralizes the centripetal force from the centre of the galaxy.

"万物负阴而抱阳,
冲气以为和"。
"Yin and Yang embrace each other, moving Qi is harmonized".
This is Lao Zi's description for Taiji. The 'S' line in the middle represents the Qi movement, balance and harmony.

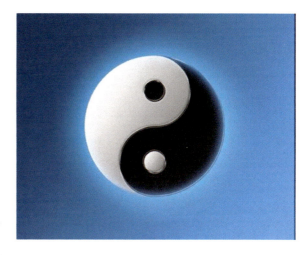

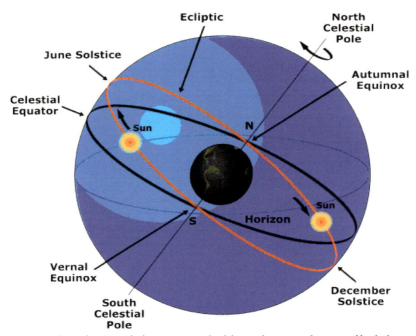

Imagine that the Earth is surrounded by a large sphere called the celestial sphere. The Earth's equator and the plane of the Earth's orbit are projected onto this sphere.

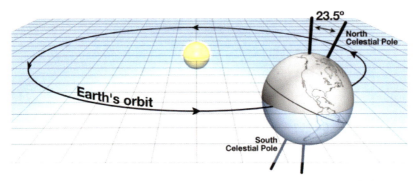

The plane of the ecliptic and the plane of the celestial equator intersect only twice a year, once on about March 21st of each year, and once on about September 22nd. The points on the celestial sphere where this occurs are called the vernal equinox and the autumnal equinox.

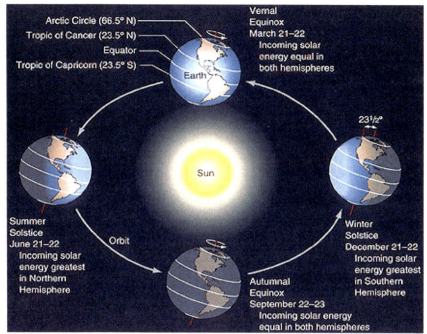

Throughout the year, the Earth is tilted at an angle of 23.5 degrees as it revolves around the Sun. Because of this, there are times when the tilt is away from the Sun and there are times when it is towards the Sun.

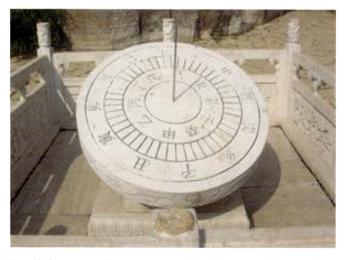

Sundial was used to measure the Yang on the earth.

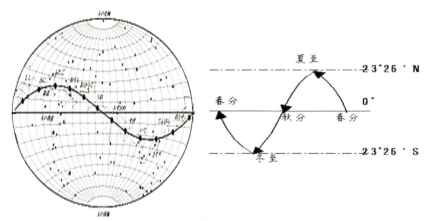

This is where the 'S' in Taiji and pre-natal Bagua came from.

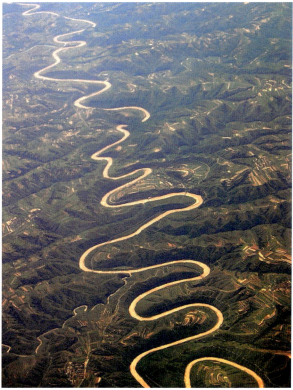

Yellow River, the Earth follows the Heaven.

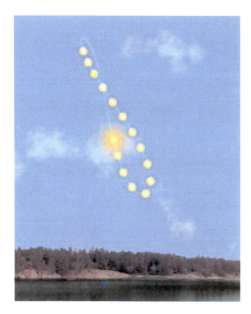

The position change of the sun in a year is in a figure 8 shape. This remind us that the 'S' in Taiji, is actually a circle.

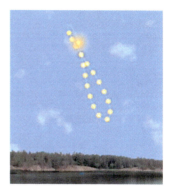

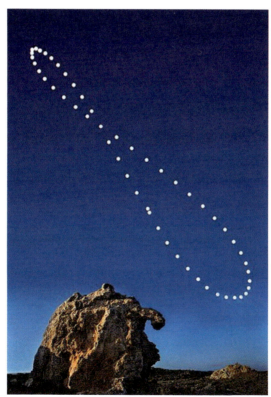

The Sun is in a figure 8 shape viewed over the four seasons

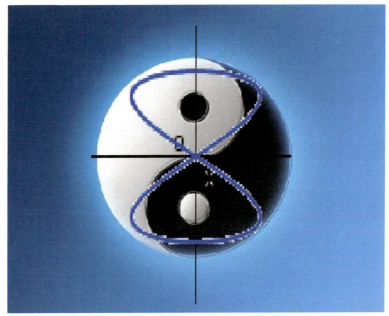

Seed Diagram of Taiji

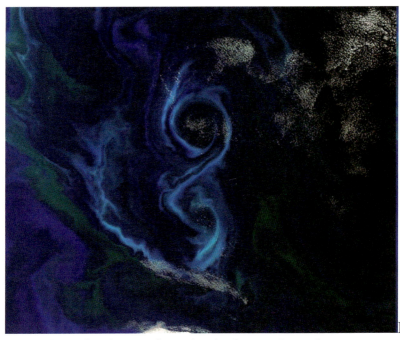Pla
nkton floating on the Atlantic Ocean shows how water
circulates in the ocean.

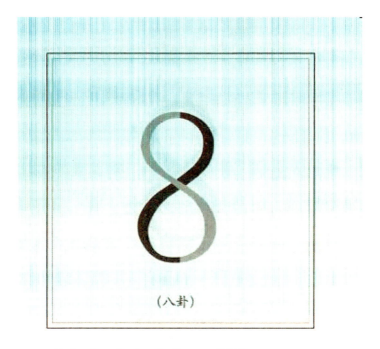

(八卦)

It is also the basic form of Qi's movement.

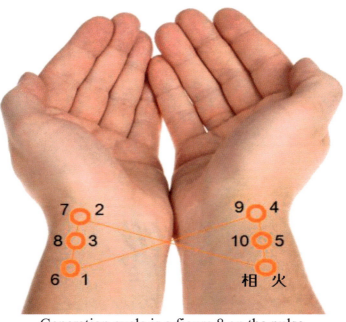

Generation cycle is a figure 8 on the pulse

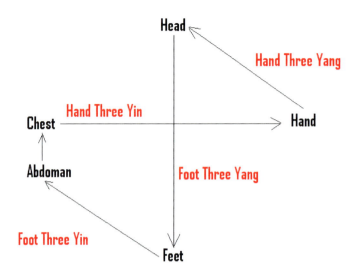

Twelve Meridian Cycle shows 8 in 3 dimensions.

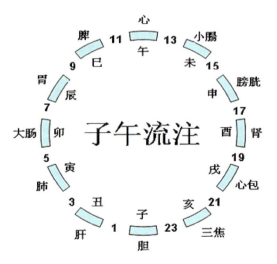

Twelve meridian cycle (Zi Wu Liu Zhu) shows a circle in 2 dimensions.

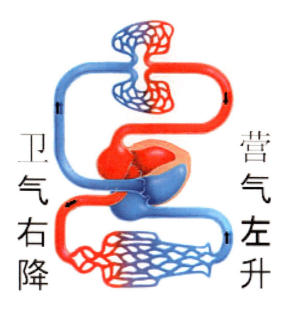

卫气右降　营气左升

It is the same for Heart Ying and Lung Wei.

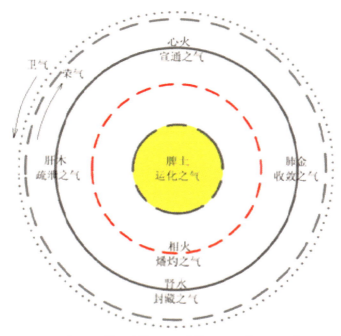

Ascending Ying and Descending Wei

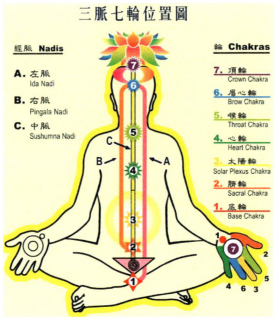

In India, there is similar description in 3 meridian and 7 circles model. There is one meridian from the top to the bottom of the trunk, known as Middle Meridian which connects to Du and Ren.

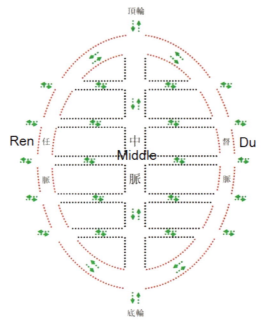

人生于地，
悬命与天，
天地合气，
命之曰人。

Human is born on the Earth, his life is designated by the heaven. The Qi from the heaven and the earth combined together, this mixed Qi is the human. Human as a whole, head on the south with the back to the sky. The back is Yang and the abdomen is Yin.

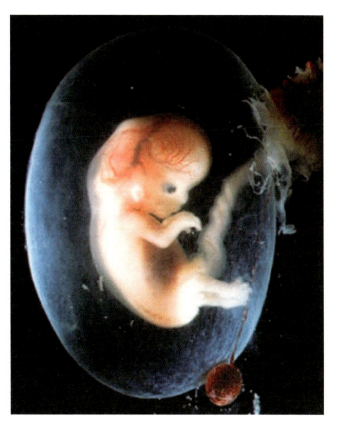

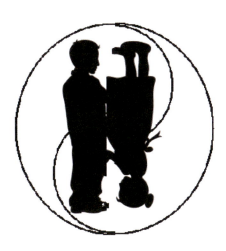

Human receive their Yin and Yang properties from Heaven and Earth. Understanding human as one Qi, the male is Yang, the female is Yin. When they combine together, they are a Taiji.

Compared to the pre-natal round and square diagram, the boy's head is Yang, the girl's head is Yang. Therefore, the back of the male is Yang, the back of the female is Yin.

Compared to the pre-natal round and square diagram, the boy's head is Yang, the girl's head is Yang. Therefore, the back of the male is Yang, the back of the female is Yin.

If both male and female have their feet on the ground, then Qi circulates in a figure 8.

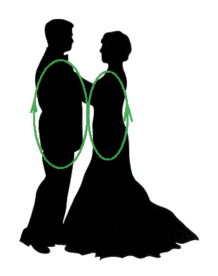

Relatively, man is Yang and woman is Yin. When facing each other, man's back faces heaven, while the woman's back faces the earth.

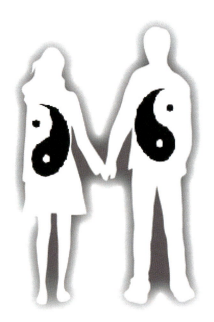

If both male and female are facing us, then the left is Yang for male and the right is Yang for female. So there is a saying: "Male left and female right" in Chinese.

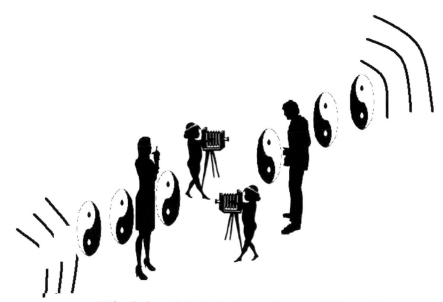

"The left and right is the pathway of Yin and Yang".

Now we know that Taiji shows differently for the same parts of the male or female body. Of course, the direction of the Qi circulation is also different.

Since the emergence of He Tu (River Gram), Chinese Medicine had its own system. Yellow Emperor developed Chinese Medicine based on experiences into a systemic medicine. The pulse regulation system in "Ling Shu" (Divine Pilot) is the brilliant model of systemic medicine.

Modern medicine has encountered bottleneck by using discrete, separate method in the journey to explore secrets of the human body and finally realized the importance of the system of human body. According to the principle of system theory, put forward the concepts of systemic biomedicine. However, in philosophy, its system still is limited compares to the Classic Chinese Medicine in which the entire system includes the Universe, Earth and Human. As of the method, it still can not shake off the shackles of mechanical materialism.

Classic Chinese medicine, found on the height of monistic ontology of Dao, summed up the common principles in the universe, Earth, and Human, applied to medicine, which catalyzed the generation of classical Chinese medicine. Since the moment of the Big Bang, the universe has produced the information and the laws, not only to control the occurrence and movement of celestial bodies, but also on the earth and human body to play a decisive role accordingly. The information and laws, summarized as Taiji in Classical Chinese Medicine, that cosmic law of motion of the double spiral structure. As a part of the whole system, all the heaven, earth and human have to follow. Therefore the requirement for being a doctor in "Inner Cannon" is "one must know the heaven above, the earth below and the human in the middle to be a doctor" because"body functions the same way as the universe and the earth."

The basic characteristics of systemic science are interlinked with the principles of "Stability", "Variability" and "Simplicity" in Yi Jing. "Stability" is to handle the specific things in the system as "one" because "one" is stable. "Variability" happens in a closely related process of a concrete practice, but this change is still in the system remains "unchanged". "Simplicity" comes from the full understanding of the principles working for the specific matters exist in a system. It made possible to simplify the universe and life phenomena beyond the complexity and is closer to the truth. "One sentence is enough for one who knows truth; one will get lost in thousands of words if you do not know the truth."

The focus for the pulse and acupuncture system in "Ling Shu" is the status of the movement of Ying (nourishing Qi) and Wei (defensive Qi). Clinically, good therapeutic results can be achieved just by regulating the pulse by acupuncture once the practitioner knows the status of Ying and Wei. Obviously, the human body is regarded as a dynamical system in "Ling Shu". The status of Ying and Wei is the status of energy conversion and distribution of the "One" Qi which is the foundation of all the body organs and functions of local processes. Therefore, the pulse and acupuncture system in "Ling Shu" guides the clinical treatment effectively for thousands of years in a way of controlling the complicity with simplicity.

"Humans were borne on the earth, their lives connected to the heaven. The Qi created by the heaven and the earth is called human." In this sense, human beings come from the Qi from the universe, so human-beings themselves are "Qi." For Chinese medicine, humans are considered as the "Qi" person first, then as the body with bone and flesh. If Qi does not circulate smoothly, it will cause illness. For treatment, the regulation of Qi, of course, is the main purpose. One must know Qi before treating Qi. The pulse is the widow of Qi, it shows acupoints for local symptoms. "Before needling, make sure always to take pulse first, give the treatment according to the Qi's movement".

Pulse diagnosis is the vital part of Classical Chinese Medicine. To know Qi by pulse is to connect the universe externally and to respond to the spirit and body internally. It connects all the parts of the body as an inseparable whole and plays an important role in controlling the local functions and process. Acupuncturists of classical style could do the treatment just by regulating the pulse because the mechanism of the pulse (here I create a new term "pulsology") is no difference to that of physiology and pathology. There are several systems of acupoints which have the functions to regulate the pulse. It can be so accurate that certain points are closely relevant to the positions of the pulse. "Doctors who are good at acupuncture should treat Yin from Yang, Yang from Yin, treat the left by needling the right, the right by needling the left, to know the other side from this side, from the surface to the internal organs, to see the hyper or hypo activity, to know the development of an illness, and then to never fail in treatment".

The manipulation of needles is to gain Qi feelings. "The importance of needling is to gain Qi feelings to get the result." So called 'Qi feelings,' are the feelings of sore, numb, distention and pain experienced of the patients. If there are no such feelings, then wait, and push Qi to come. When Qi comes, doctors have to tell if it is a bad Qi or a good Qi. "A bad Qi will feel tight and rapid, while a good Qi feels smooth and slow". Then do the acupuncture technique of tonification or discharge accordingly. Good Qi can be made stronger by tonification and bad Qi can be released by discharge. "Acupuncture is all about the reversing and following of the Qi, and harmonizing it."

Tonification and discharging technique are based on the following or reversing Qi. Mal-manipulation may happen if one does not know the local Qi's movement. Qi exists everywhere, out and in everywhere and up and down everywhere. Male and female are different in terms morning or afternoon, left or right. It is variability. Nevertheless, Ying and Wei follow the routine of the sun and the moon, this is stability on macro sense. It is "Simplicity" for "Ling Shu" to regulate Qi by regulating the pulse with only one or two needles to gain instant result for the local symptoms. "Doctors who are not skillful enough focus on the body, while good doctors focus on the Qi".

Because of the deep understanding of the disease and the clinical use of pulse diagnosis, practioners in ancient times were able to gain insight into the mystery of human life, causing a great revolution of medical science, which led to the golden age of Chinese Medicine in Han and Tang Dynasties. Till today, the highly developed modern medicine still can not compare to the brilliant achievements of the ancient Chinese medicine in terms of human understanding at holistic level. Those good ones, who know the pulse differentiation at that time, could cure nine out of ten with confidence. Besides, "the results come as quick as the sound from a beaten drum". This shows that the prevailing medical practice had been out of blindness and avoided subjective arbitrary to some extent.

Unfortunately, all of this for us nowadays, seems to be dreams from our previous life. Modern Chinese medicine can not reproduce all of those; can not understand all of those; got lost in both direction and confidence. As if these glorious achievements never happened in the history of Chinese medicine. The later declination of modern Chinese medicine is not just due to the depreciation of pulse diagnosis, but the lost of the main systemic holistic concepts. The holistic concept is the soul of classic Chinese medicine and is its superiority. Chinese Medicine could only rediscover "itself" reflected the history, go back to the classical way and then, it can strive out of the woods and reproduce the brilliance.

# ABOUT THE AUTHOR
## Joe Ranallo

Dr. Xiaochuan Pan, the founder and owner of Pan's Clinic in Victoria, BC, brings to Canada an impressive academic and career resume. He holds a Bachelor of Medicine (1983) from the Heilongjiang University of TCM. In 1990, he was awarded a Master in Microbiology and Immunology from the prestigious Dalian Medical University. From 1990 to 1999, he worked as a professional researcher funded by the central Government of China. As part of this appointment, Dr. Pan founded and directed the Dalian Institute of Integrative Medicine that blends traditional and modern Medicine. Since moving to Canada in 2000, Dr. Pan has practiced and taught TCM. He has managed clinics in Victoria, Nanaimo, and Sydney, BC and has offered courses and workshops in Vancouver Island and the Lower Mainland. He has been a frequent keynote speaker at BC TCM related functions and is often invited to play his Erhu and Guzheng, or double stringed Chinese violin and Chinese harp, of which he is a virtuoso. The US based International Institute of Holistic Medicine profiles Dr. Pan as one its Canadian TCM experts. In 2013, this Institute honors 15 Canadian TCM practitioners, only four of which are based in BC. Dr. Pan has certainly earned a position of distinction among Canada's TCM experts. This is Dr. Pan the resume. There is also Dr. Pan the person.

As the previous paragraph implies, Dr. Pan is a committed researcher and learner. Several times a year, he flies back to China to remain current on the latest discoveries in TCM. He is especially drawn to the latest findings on the Pulses and on the earliest records of TCM literature. His considerable knowledge is amplified with each of his trips. Each time he returns, he seems far more intelligent than when he left. Sometimes I questions where he has gone and wonder if, instead of going to China, he has boarded some space ship where superior alien beings from some distant galaxy have modified his DNA and raised his brain to a higher frequency of consciousness. He is so well informed about the stars, planets, and galaxies that I sometimes wonder if he has actually been there.

He is not only an exceptional scholar, he is also an inspiring instructor. His students respect and venerate him. They value his in- depth preparation and trust his extensive knowledge which he shares freely. They are particularly impressed with the multitude of visuals he uses. When Dr. Pan did not have sufficient students to offer an innovative extra curricular course on Yi Jing, Level 1, one of the students took on the responsibility to find more candidates. Dr. Pan is one of the most sought out teachers in the BC TCM community.

Dr. Pan is an esteemed innovator. He has introduced Canada to some unique therapies. He has brought us the Transdermal Herbal Patches that he calls acupuncture without needles. He has not only taught his students to use the patches properly, but has also devised a system of his own in which he uses the patches to rebalance the pulses. He has also introduced the Floating Needle technique which successfully relieves pain issues in one to three sessions. He has also devised an herbal remedy strategy of his own in which patients ingest predetermined doses of Traditional Chinese formulas at daybreak and at night. Most importantly, he has learned to use boiled herbs to successfully treat serious, life threatening illnesses. These are some of the innovations Dr. Pan has introduced since he arrived in Canada at the turn of the millennium.

Because he has access to a variety of treatments, he is able to offer his patients something that they really value and appreciate-- the element of choice. After diagnosing their imbalances, Dr. Pan lays out for the patients a variety of ways of rebalancing them. He then let's the patients choose the treatment protocols they want. By so doing, he is inviting the patients become part of the cure.

This, in a nutshell, is a miniature introduction to who this remarkable Dr. Pan is and to the wonderful service he provides for humanity. We are fortunate and blessed to have him among us.

# References

Many pictures were from internet through google search. I try my best to list the links to show the sources. If there were authors I missed to mention, please e-mail me to dr.pan.xiaochuan@gmail.com.

1. https://www.youtube.com/watch?v=17jymDn0W6U

2. http://www.youtube.com/watch?v=xp-8HysWkxw

3. http://esophoria.org/

4. http://aflam-muusiiiiiiiiiiiiiiic.blogspot.ca

5. http://causeyourlife.com/2010/08/crop-circle-july-25-2010/

6. Wikipedia, the free encyclopedia

Made in the USA
Charleston, SC
24 October 2013